T0146361

Military Behavioral Health Staff Perspectives on Telehealth Following the Onset of the COVID-19 Pandemic

KIMBERLY A. HEPNER, JESSICA L. SOUSA, JUSTIN HUMMER, HAROLD ALAN PINCUS, RYAN ANDREW BROWN

Prepared for the Defense Health Agency
Approved for public release; distribution unlimited

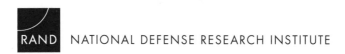 NATIONAL DEFENSE RESEARCH INSTITUTE

For more information on this publication, visit **www.rand.org/t/RRA421-2**.

About RAND

The RAND Corporation is a research organization that develops solutions to public policy challenges to help make communities throughout the world safer and more secure, healthier and more prosperous. RAND is nonprofit, nonpartisan, and committed to the public interest. To learn more about RAND, visit www.rand.org.

Research Integrity

Our mission to help improve policy and decisionmaking through research and analysis is enabled through our core values of quality and objectivity and our unwavering commitment to the highest level of integrity and ethical behavior. To help ensure our research and analysis are rigorous, objective, and nonpartisan, we subject our research publications to a robust and exacting quality-assurance process; avoid both the appearance and reality of financial and other conflicts of interest through staff training, project screening, and a policy of mandatory disclosure; and pursue transparency in our research engagements through our commitment to the open publication of our research findings and recommendations, disclosure of the source of funding of published research, and policies to ensure intellectual independence. For more information, visit www.rand.org/about/principles.

RAND's publications do not necessarily reflect the opinions of its research clients and sponsors.

Published by the RAND Corporation, Santa Monica, Calif.
© 2021 RAND Corporation
RAND® is a registered trademark.

Library of Congress Cataloging-in-Publication Data is available for this publication.
ISBN: 978-1-9774-0825-9

About This Report

The Military Health System (MHS), like other health care systems, needed to pivot quickly in response to the COVID-19 pandemic to minimize disruptions in care for its beneficiaries. At the same time the MHS was facing operational challenges to delivering behavioral health (BH) care, increased distress related to the pandemic may have driven higher demand for BH care among service members and their dependents. For service members who receive care through the MHS for posttraumatic stress disorder, depression, or substance use disorder, telehealth offers a potentially promising alternative when in-person visits are not feasible. However, prior to the pandemic, telehealth use was low across the MHS.

Between July and October 2020, RAND Corporation researchers interviewed staff who delivered or oversaw BH care at military treatment facilities to determine the extent to which MHS providers had used telehealth with these patients since the onset of the pandemic, what their experiences and concerns were, and what gaps or barriers needed to be addressed to expand the use of telehealth across the MHS. These findings subsequently informed recommendations to help the MHS continue to integrate telehealth in a way that meets the BH needs of service members.

The research reported here was completed in March 2021 and underwent security review with the Defense Office of Prepublication and Security Review before public release.

RAND National Security Research Division

This research was sponsored by the Defense Health Agency and conducted within the Forces and Resources Policy Center of the RAND National Security Research Division (NSRD), which operates the National Defense Research Institute (NDRI), a federally funded research and development center sponsored by the Office of the Secretary of Defense, the Joint Staff, the Unified Combatant Commands, the Navy, the Marine Corps, the defense agencies, and the defense intelligence enterprise.

For more information on the RAND Forces and Resources Policy Center, see www.rand.org/nsrd/frp or contact the director (contact information is provided on the webpage).

Acknowledgments

We gratefully acknowledge the support of our project sponsor, Robert Ciulla, Connected Health Branch, Clinical Support Division, Medical Affairs, Defense Health Agency. We also appreciate the ongoing support we received from Anju Bhargava, Fuad Issa, Kate McGraw, and staff at the Connected Health Branch and the Psychological Health Center of Excellence. We appreciate the valuable insights we received from our reviewers, Craig Rosen and Lori Uscher-Pines. We addressed their constructive critiques as part of RAND's rigorous quality assurance process to improve the quality of this report. We thank Lauren Skrabala for her contributions to sections of this report, Rosa Maria Torres for her assistance in preparing the report, and Jessica Sousa for overseeing human subjects and regulatory approvals for the project. Finally, we extend our gratitude to the providers and administrators who participated in project interviews and personnel at each military treatment facility who collaborated with us on recruitment.

Summary

The COVID-19 pandemic prompted sweeping changes to behavioral health (BH) care delivery, and the Military Health System (MHS) faced challenges similar to those of other health care systems. The MHS needed to minimize disruptions and ensure continuity of BH care for service members, leading to a rapid increase in the use of telehealth. The objectives of the work presented in this report were to assess the perspectives and experiences of military BH staff regarding their use of telehealth following the onset of the pandemic. The findings informed recommendations to guide the MHS in better integrating telehealth into BH care. We interviewed staff who delivered or oversaw BH care at military treatment facilities (MTFs) between July and October 2020 to help the MHS assess how these facilities and individual providers adapted to providing BH care in the midst of a pandemic, their experiences with telehealth as a BH care delivery method, and the feasibility of using telehealth for this type of care in the post-pandemic future.

The COVID-19 Pandemic May Have Increased Demand for Behavioral Health Care in the MHS

Posttraumatic stress disorder (PTSD), depression, and substance use disorders (SUDs) are all common among U.S. service members. Prior RAND Corporation research analyzing MHS administrative data identified several differences in BH care access and quality across service members with these conditions. Specifically, access to and receipt of recommended BH care was generally found to be lower among reserve-component service members than active-duty service members and lower among service members who lived in areas remote from an MTF compared with those who lived near such a facility (Hummer et al., 2021; Hepner et al., 2021; Hepner et al., 2017). The MHS aims to provide high-quality care for service members with BH conditions, and the recommendations from those studies—which included the increased use of telehealth—highlighted opportunities to address these differences and ensure that all service members receive the BH treatment they need.

However, the pandemic may have affected MHS efforts to improve service members' access to BH care and the quality of care they received. At the same time, increased distress related to the pandemic may have increased demand for BH care among service members and their dependents who are eligible for TRICARE. Nationally representative longitudinal survey data from the Centers for Disease Control and Prevention and RAND showed sharp increases in mental health symptoms and psychological distress as a result of the pandemic (Breslau et al., 2021; Czeisler et al., 2020), particularly among younger adults and racial/ethnic minorities. Preliminary data suggest that this trend held true for service members as well: A survey conducted from March to May 2020 found that 15 percent of active-duty service members experienced worsening symptoms of an existing anxiety or depressive disorder diagnosis (Strong, Akin, and Brazer, 2020). Another 18 percent reported experiencing anxiety or depressive symptoms with no preexisting diagnosis, suggesting new onset of these symptoms.

Telehealth for Behavioral Health Care in the MHS

In the MHS, *telehealth* has been defined as "the use of technology to provide health care consultation, education, assessment, treatment, care coordination and support for health care providers and patients separated by distance" (MHS, undated).[1] The MHS has used telehealth—whether real-time interaction (synchronous) or non-simultaneous information exchanges between patients and providers (asynchronous)—for more than 20 years. It has been used for numerous conditions, but its most common application has been for BH care. There are many different models of telehealth, but most have similar benefits, including convenience for patients who need to schedule appointments around work and child care obligations. Telehealth can also increase access to BH care for service members who live in remote areas or require care in deployed settings. Research also suggests that telehealth is an effective means of care delivery for PTSD, depression,

---

[1] Although other terms can be used (e.g., *virtual health, virtual behavioral health, telebehavioral health*), we use *telehealth* throughout this report because that was the terminology used in our interviews with BH staff.

and SUDs. For the MHS, telehealth has the potential to address surges in demand for BH care, provided that procedures are in place to flexibly reassign workloads across providers or care teams and to overcome challenges associated with a shortage of BH care providers.

Prior to the pandemic, telehealth use was low in the MHS: A RAND study of MHS administrative data found that less than 3 percent of service members treated for PTSD, depression, or SUD in 2016–2017 received synchronous (real-time) telehealth care (Hepner et al., 2021).

Interview Sample Selection and Methods

We interviewed 53 BH staff at ten MTFs. We identified facilities and staff to interview using a tiered stratified sampling approach. First, we selected MTFs to maximize variation by service branch; geographical location; proportion of BH visits by remote service members being treated for PTSD, depression, and SUDs; MTF size; quality of BH care; and types of telehealth services offered by the MTFs. The distribution included slightly more Army MTFs, larger MTFs, and MTFs offering higher-quality BH care. We then selected staff to interview using the following eligibility criteria: (1) a member of the U.S. military (Army, Navy, Air Force, or Marine Corps) in the active component, in the National Guard/reserve (active-duty or active status), or a government/U.S. Department of Defense civilian and (2) a provider or administrator who delivered or oversaw care at an MTF for service members with at least one of the target diagnoses (PTSD, depression, or SUD).[2] A mix of provider types—including psychiatrists, psychologists, master's-level counselors, substance use counselors, and primary care practitioners—helped us capture a wide range of experiences with BH care delivery and telehealth.

We conducted interviews by phone or via a secure web-based videoconferencing platform between July and October 2020. The interviews used a semistructured protocol to collect details on providers' use of telehealth following the onset of the COVID-19 pandemic, organizational and clinical

---

[2] Contracted staff were excluded because it was not feasible within the scope of our project to meet the additional regulatory requirements to include them.

factors associated with the use of telehealth, perspectives on patient satisfaction and the need for provider and patient familiarization with telehealth, and experiences providing telehealth to remote service members.

Key Findings

Use of Telehealth Increased Dramatically Following the Onset of the Pandemic, but It Varied Within and Across MTFs, and Many MTFs Were Already Returning to In-Person Care

Nearly all respondents noted a dramatic shift from in-person care to audio-only or video telehealth or to a combination of in-person and telehealth modalities early in the pandemic. Some described using audio-only telehealth for shorter visits or "check-ins," while others mentioned attempting to deliver full-length psychotherapy sessions. More than half reported at least some integration of mobile apps into their BH care delivery. There was variation across sites and between providers in the proportion of telehealth visits relative to in-person care during the pandemic. At the time of our interviews, half of respondents across all MTFs told us they were getting "back to normal" and seeing more patients in person.

Most Providers Were Open to Using Video Telehealth, but Widespread Technological Challenges and a Lack of Clear Policy Guidance Impeded More-Frequent Use

Nearly all providers were using audio-only telehealth at the time of our interviews, yet only about a quarter indicated that they were open to continuing to use it. Most were not yet using video telehealth; among those who did, just over half indicated that they were open to continuing to use it. Overall, more than three-quarters expressed an interest in using video telehealth in the future. Reasons for low uptake of video telehealth included administrative and technological barriers, such as insufficient internet bandwidth and equipment, difficulty accessing telehealth platforms while teleworking, a lack of technical support, and concerns about reliability and data security. Staff at most MTFs also expressed frustration with bureaucratic barriers, unclear guidance, or a perceived lack of support for telehealth at the MTF or Defense Health Agency (DHA) level.

Staff Expressed Concerns About Using Telehealth with High-Risk Patients, Those Diagnosed with PTSD or SUD, and Those Receiving Group Therapy

Nearly all respondents shared opinions about the appropriateness of telehealth for specific patient populations. Around half expressed concerns about using telehealth—particularly audio-only telehealth—to treat high-risk patients or patients with high symptom severity. Reasons given included an inability to accurately assess certain symptoms. Most staff reported that high-risk patients were typically seen in person during the pandemic. In addition, nearly one-third and one-fifth, respectively, expressed some concern about using telehealth with any patient with PTSD or SUD. About one-quarter of respondents mentioned that group therapy sessions had stopped since the onset of the pandemic, and about one-fifth expressed concerns about using telehealth to deliver group therapy. Across nearly all MTFs, around one-third of respondents shared concerns about using telehealth to conduct intake assessments or suggested that it should be used with established patients only.

Staff Indicated That Both Patients and Providers Needed More Orientation to Telehealth

Just over half of BH staff reported that they believed patients liked telehealth, largely citing greater convenience. However, nearly one-third reported that some patients *disliked* telehealth and preferred to receive care in person. Reasons included a lack of trust in the technology or difficulty using it. Some staff described a "learning curve" for both providers and patients as they became more comfortable with telehealth modalities.

Staff Believed That Telehealth Was a Promising Approach for Service Members Who Lived Far from an MTF, but They Reported Barriers to Using Telehealth with These Patients

The majority of BH staff reported that they did not use telehealth with remote service members prior to the pandemic, and nearly half said that telehealth was not always used with this population during the pandemic. More than half acknowledged the unique value of telehealth for these service members, including increased access and continuity of care. Although most said that telehealth had ameliorated barriers for one or more remote service member patients, there was broad recognition that existing MTF staffing levels and referral practices did not support ongoing use of tele-health with this population. Respondents also cited concerns about treating high-risk or high-symptom-severity patients as a possible barrier.

Recommendations

The following recommendations can help the MHS continue to integrate telehealth to meet the BH needs of service members and guide decision-making regarding policies and practices for the adoption of telehealth for BH care at an enterprise scale.

Recommendation 1. Develop Policy Guidance on the Use of Telehealth for Patients with Specific BH Conditions

DHA released interim guidance on data security and privacy in March and August 2020 (Place, 2020; Cordts, 2020), along with standards of practice for BH during the pandemic period (DHA, 2020), but, as of March 2021, there was no formal procedural instruction for telehealth. Policy guidance should address both the technological requirements and expectations for high-quality treatment delivery via telehealth. It might also be worthwhile to standardize policy guidance with clinical guidelines on the safe treat-ment of patients with various clinical issues. Allowances might be made for MTF- or command-level variation in telehealth implementation while still establishing minimum legal and regulatory requirements at the system level.

Recommendation 2. Develop and Implement a Strategic Plan to Ensure That Providers Have Adequate Technology to Support Video Telehealth

Across all the MTFs in our study, staff reported technological infrastructure barriers to telehealth adoption—including a lack of adequate technology to allow video telehealth, poor connectivity, inadequate bandwidth, and diffi-culty using telehealth platforms. It appears that the MHS would benefit from a strategic plan to address these limitations. Ideally, the MHS would adopt a user-friendly, reliable, and secure audio-only and video telehealth platform that is compatible with multiple types of devices; interoperable with GENESIS, the electronic medical record system being deployed across MTFs; and adaptable to both individual and group treatment. It might be beneficial to first evaluate existing platforms and identify potential improvements to meet these needs.

Recommendation 3. Provide Clinical and Technical Training on the Use of Telehealth

Recommendation 3a. Provide Training on the Clinical Aspects of Telehealth

Staff expressed concerns about using telehealth in a variety of clinical situations (e.g., with high-risk patients), suggesting a need for additional training on the clinical aspects of telehealth. Training that targets providers' specific concerns and competency levels would increase comfort, knowledge, and skills and would potentially improve attitudes toward telehealth. Providers also need standardized, empirically based guidance to identify which patients are appropriate candidates for telehealth, how to assess patients and deliver evidence-based psychotherapy using telehealth, and how to respond when there are concerns about patient safety. They would also benefit from materials to socialize patients to telehealth.

Recommendation 3b. Provide Technical Training and Support for Telehealth

Staff expressed a desire for access to technical support and training specific to telehealth implementation. Training on the technological elements of telehealth modalities and best practices for interacting with patients this way could help mitigate this barrier. It might be worthwhile to identify existing technical support staff and conduct an initial assessment of potential scalability at a given MTF. At the system level, it may be useful to increase information technology staffing to ensure that someone is on site at each MTF to troubleshoot or provide in-home assistance (for providers who are teleworking).

Conclusions

Preliminary evidence indicates that the COVID-19 pandemic increased demand for BH care among service members, just as it did for civilian populations. Furthermore, pandemic-related restrictions affected the ability to deliver BH care to service members in person. Telehealth filled a gap for some MTFs and providers early on in the pandemic, but there was some uncertainty about its future utility at the time of our interviews. The findings and recommendations in this report illustrate how telehealth can—with the appropriate training, technology, guidance, and policies—increase access to BH care and help the MHS meet the needs of all service members.

Contents

Figure and Tables

Figure

Tables

CHAPTER ONE

Introduction

The Military Health System (MHS) aims to support overall military readiness by providing timely access to high-quality care for service members with behavioral health (BH) conditions. Beginning in March 2020, the COVID-19 pandemic significantly disrupted U.S. health care delivery, and the MHS needed to ensure that service members who needed BH care could receive treatment uninterrupted. The restrictions on in-person care delivery presented opportunities to use telehealth to meet these needs. As the pandemic progressed, there were questions in the health care sector about whether telehealth was here to stay. The objectives of the work presented in this report were to assess the perspectives and experiences of military BH staff regarding their use of telehealth following the onset of the pandemic. The findings informed recommendations to guide the MHS in better integrating telehealth into BH care. We interviewed BH staff who delivered or oversaw BH care at military treatment facilities (MTFs) between July and October 2020 to help the MHS assess how these facilities and individual providers adapted to providing BH care in the midst of a pandemic, their experiences with telehealth as a BH care delivery method, and the feasibility of using telehealth for this type of care in the post-pandemic future.

This chapter provides an overview of MHS care for service members with BH conditions and explores the role of telehealth in BH care.

Meeting the Behavioral Health Needs of Service Members

BH conditions, including posttraumatic stress disorder (PTSD), depression, and substance use disorders (SUDs), are common among service members.

A meta-analysis of ten studies reported prevalence estimates of 7.1 percent for depression, 8.9 percent for PTSD, and 11.7 percent for alcohol use disorders among active-duty service members (Cohen et al., 2015). The 2018 U.S. Department of Defense (DoD) Health-Related Behaviors Survey of active-component service members found similar prevalence rates across the service branches: 10.5 percent for probable PTSD and 16.6 percent for serious psychological distress (e.g., depression and anxiety) (Meadows et al., 2021). On that survey, 34.0 percent of military personnel reported heavy episodic drinking (five or more drinks on one occasion for men, or four or more for women, at least once in the previous month), and 9.9 percent were heavy drinkers (engaging in heavy episodic drinking on five or more days in the previous month) (Meadows et al., 2021).

The MHS aims to provide high-quality care for service members with BH conditions, but recent research has highlighted areas for improvement. In August 2020, DoD's Office of Inspector General reported that service members and their families did not have timely access to BH services, either though MTFs or community providers contracted through TRICARE. For example, in a review of six-month appointment and referral data from 13 MTFs, the office found that seven MTFs or their private-sector care network providers and facilities did not meet the standard for specialty BH care access each month. Fifty-three percent of active-duty service members and their families in the TRICARE East and West regions who needed BH care and were referred to private-sector care did not receive care. At nine of 13 MTFs, patients' follow-up treatment may have been delayed or was not otherwise provided in accordance with established standards (Defense Health Agency [DHA] Procedural Instruction 6490.02, 2018). In response, the American Psychological Association submitted an urgent call for DoD to address the report's recommendations and improve access to BH care (Evans, 2020).

Prior RAND Corporation research comprehensively assessed service members' access to care and the quality of care they received for PTSD, depression, or SUD through the MHS in 2016–2017 (Hepner et al., 2021; Hummer et al., 2021). The study extended to service members who lived in areas that were *remote* from an MTF, defined as living in a zip code that made the service member eligible for TRICARE Prime Remote status. These service members may face additional challenges accessing high-quality care.

In fact, across most domains assessed, remote service members were less likely to receive recommended BH care, including psychotherapy, follow-up visits after initiating new medication treatment, and outpatient follow-up after discharge from a psychiatric hospitalization (Hepner et al., 2021). The study's findings regarding access to care were consistent with those of the DoD Office of Inspector General. The research team, like others, recommended that the MHS expand its use of telehealth to better meet the BH needs of service members (Hummer et al., 2021; Brown et al., 2015).

Impact of the COVID-19 Pandemic on the Need for Behavioral Health Care

Early evidence suggests that there has been an increase in BH needs since the onset of the COVID-19 pandemic. The Centers for Disease Control and Prevention reported a threefold increase in anxiety disorder symptoms and a fourfold increase in the prevalence of depressive disorder among U.S. adults, along with elevated suicidal ideation and increased substance use compared with pre-pandemic levels—with young adults and racial/ethnic minorities being disproportionately affected (Czeisler et al., 2020). Similarly, results from nationally representative surveys have revealed a sharp increase in both the frequency and amount of alcohol consumption (Pollard, Tucker, and Green, 2020) and a tripling in the prevalence of depressive symptoms (Ettman et al., 2020) and "serious psychological distress" (McGinty et al., 2020). A RAND study found that equal numbers of people experienced serious psychological distress in a 30-day period during the pandemic as did so over an entire year prior to the pandemic (Breslau et al., 2021).

Preliminary survey data suggest that service members have been similarly affected. On a survey conducted between March and May 2020, 15 percent of active-duty service members said they had experienced worsened symptoms of an existing anxiety or depressive disorder diagnosis (Strong, Akin, and Brazer, 2020). Another 18 percent reported experiencing anxiety or depressive symptoms with no preexisting diagnosis, suggesting new onset of these symptoms. Although it was a non-probability survey and therefore not necessarily representative of the general service member population, these findings suggest that there were some increases in service members' BH needs since the onset of the pandemic.

The pandemic had a marked effect on MHS operations, leading to a temporary "pause" in the transition to DHA oversight of all care delivery, a major transformative effort mandated by the National Defense Authorization Act for Fiscal Year 2017 (Pub. L. 114-328, Sec. 702). The pause was lifted in November 2020, with the five regional "markets" (Colorado; Hawaii; Puget Sound, Washington; San Antonio, Texas; and Tidewater, Virginia) beginning their transition in December 2020 (MHS Communications Office, 2021). Despite the pause in the transition, the pandemic may also have presented the MHS with an opportunity to rapidly increase its use of telehealth (MHS Communications Office, 2020).

Telehealth for Behavioral Health Care in the Military Health System

In the MHS, *telehealth* is defined as "the use of technology to provide health care consultation, education, assessment, treatment, care coordination and support for health care providers and patients separated by distance" (MHS, undated). Examples of other terms for telehealth include *virtual health* and *telemedicine*. When *telehealth* is used in support of a particular clinical area, the term often references the clinical area (e.g., *telebehavioral health, teleradiology*). As with the more general terms, *telebehavioral health* and *virtual behavioral health* are interchangeable. For the purposes of this report, and to be consistent with the terminology in our interviews with BH staff, we use the term *telehealth* to denote the use of telebehavioral or virtual BH tools. Synchronous telehealth involves real-time patient-provider interactive audio-only or video communications, while asynchronous telehealth involves non-simultaneous exchange of information or records via email or mobile applications for home-based symptom management or tracking.

Utility of Telehealth for Behavioral Health Care

Telehealth is an effective means of care delivery for PTSD (Acierno et al., 2017; Bolton and Dorstyn, 2015; Varker et al., 2019), depression (Berryhill et al., 2019; Varker et al., 2019), and SUDs (Benavides-Vaello, Strode, and Sheeran, 2013; King et al., 2009; Santa Ana et al., 2013). Specifically, research indicates that psychotherapy conducted via video telehealth is as effective as face-to-face sessions in treating a wide range of BH conditions, with studies typically demonstrating high strength, positive direction, high consistency, moderate to high generalizability (given that many studies focus solely on veteran populations), and high applicability and patient satisfaction (Bashshur et al., 2016; Greenbaum, 2020; Gros et al., 2013; Morland et al., 2020).

The evidence for audio-only telehealth is less robust than for video telehealth. Fewer studies have evaluated the effectiveness of audio-only telehealth in diverse treatment settings, with a variety of patient characteristics, and using controlled treatment designs with in-person comparison groups. There is clear evidence for its effectiveness in treating depression and supporting smoking cessation when compared with minimal or no intervention. Preliminary evidence also supports audio-only telehealth as equivalent to in-person care for depression and anxiety disorders (Coughtrey and Pistrang, 2018; Lovell et al., 2006; Mohr et al., 2012; Rosen et al., 2021). More research regarding the effectiveness of audio-only telehealth in addressing other problems (e.g., PTSD, psychiatric management) is needed, and it remains an open question whether audio-only telehealth is generally as effective as video telehealth for various conditions. Finally, asynchronous telehealth, through the use of mobile applications and websites, assists both self-care and symptom monitoring to improve ongoing care management (DoD, 2019).

The convenience of telehealth can also increase access to care. For example, telehealth eliminates travel time for patients and reduces conflicts with work schedules (MHS, undated). One group that could benefit the most from telehealth are service members who reside remotely from an MTF, especially when such care in not readily available in the surrounding community. In deployed settings, telehealth can reduce the need for providers and service members to travel, potentially reducing costs and manpower to facilitate such transfers (Pamplin et al., 2019; DoD, 2019; Waibel et al., 2017). In addition, telehealth can reduce the stigma associated with going into a clinic that offers BH care (MHS, undated; Stoyanov et al., 2015; DoD, 2019).

Telehealth is a useful delivery tool for ongoing BH treatment. In addition to reducing some access barriers, such as transportation and distance, it can be used on a "surge" basis to meet increased demand for services (DoD, 2019). However, telehealth does not necessarily reduce access barriers related to provider supply (or clinical workload).

The United States is facing a shortage of BH providers, including psychiatrists, psychologists, and nurses (Health Resources and Services Administration, 2020), and this extends to the MHS, where the trend is exacerbated by competition with the private and public sectors and limited awareness of DoD educational programs for the health professions (Pub. L. 116-92, 2019). The capacity to realize telehealth's benefits and meet patient demand will depend, in part, on the ability to recruit and retain sufficient numbers of BH providers. Such efforts are ongoing within the MHS (Pub. L. 116-92, 2019). At the MHS enterprise level, telehealth has the potential to improve workflows and reduce the impact of workforce shortages by strengthening partnerships between BH clinics at MTFs and optimizing existing capacity in response to demand. For example, "hub-and-spoke" telehealth delivery models involve a provider at a centralized clinic who delivers care to patients at outlying satellite clinics. Review studies by the U.S. Department of Veterans Affairs (VA) have shown that this model of telehealth delivery is a feasible, acceptable, cost-effective, and clinically effective alternative to in-person therapies (Lindsay et al., 2017; Morland et al., 2017; Turgoose, Ashwick, and Murphy, 2018). The Air Force developed a regional hub-and-spoke model for telehealth care delivery (DoD, 2019), while a similar model piloted by the Navy was found to be a cost-effective method of reducing the need for civilian referrals and medical evacuations (Lin et al., 2017). For administrators and providers, increased use of telehealth can improve interdisciplinary teams' screening efficiency, referral tracking, and consultation services to better coordinate care (Docherty et al., 2020).

The Use of Telehealth for Behavioral Health Care in the MHS

While telehealth has been used in the MHS for more than 20 years, efforts to expand its integration continue. In fiscal years 2016 and 2017, BH care represented the majority of direct care and private-sector synchronous telehealth provided to TRICARE beneficiaries (DoD, 2019). However, a RAND study of care for PTSD, depression, and SUD in the MHS in 2016–2017 found that less than 3 percent of service members received synchronous telehealth (Hepner et al., 2021), according to administrative treatment data. The RAND report recommended that the MHS increase its use of synchronous telehealth and identified telehealth as an approach to improve care for remote service members. In 2015, the MHS chartered a telehealth workgroup, the Virtual Health Work Group, to coordinate and move telehealth forward at the MHS enterprise level. Subsequently, as part of its 2018 MHS Virtual Health Strategic Plan, the group identified multiple opportunities for expansion, including in synchronous, asynchronous, and remote health monitoring capabilities (DoD, 2019).[1]

According to a DoD report to Congress, successful widespread implementation of telehealth will require addressing substantial challenges (DoD, 2019). The MHS will need technological infrastructure with adequate capacity to support telehealth that is user-friendly for both providers and patients. Its Virtual Health Strategic Plan sets the stage to fully integrate telehealth into information technology (IT) infrastructure planning, which includes translating functional (clinical) requirements into technical requirements and acquiring and sustaining a formal telehealth platform. Administrators and providers will need training to ensure that they and their patients understand how to access and use telehealth technologies. Providers will need additional training and continuing education to ensure compliance in delivering certain forms of evidence-based care via telehealth. Organizational issues, such as workflows and financial management, are also important components of a larger-scale telehealth initiative.

In addition to the challenges outlined in the 2019 report to Congress, it will be important to consider personal data security, confidentiality, and patient safety. Increased use of telehealth will require significant planning and financial investment. Although all sectors that rely on technology face similar challenges, the stakes are particularly high for the MHS, which plays a critical role in force readiness and safeguarding national security.

---

[1] The Virtual Health Work Group has since been replaced by the Virtual Health Advisory Board and the Virtual Health Coordinating Group.

Telehealth for Behavioral Health Care During the COVID-19 Pandemic

Amid a surge in cases of COVID-19, major disruptions to the delivery of BH services, and increased BH care needs, the U.S. government and health systems across the United States raced to adopt policies to increase telehealth uptake and reduce the need for physical meetings between patients and providers (Chen et al., 2020; Kola, 2020; Webster, 2020; Zhang, Boden, and Trafton, 2021). On March 17, 2020, the federal government announced a temporary 60-day relaxation of Health Insurance Portability and Accountability Act (HIPAA) security rules to permit telehealth via nonsecure platforms. Less than two weeks later, the Centers for Medicare and Medicaid Services issued "an unprecedented array of temporary regulatory waivers and new rules to equip the American healthcare system with maximum flexibility to respond to the 2019 Novel Coronavirus (COVID-19) pandemic" (Centers for Medicare and Medicaid Services, 2020), allowing for more than 80 additional services to be delivered via telehealth. These measures included allowances for audio-only telehealth for BH counseling.

Across the civilian health care sector, there were significant increases in the use of telehealth, and much of the growth during early phases of the pandemic was driven by BH care visits (Uscher-Pines et al., 2020). As the pandemic continued into May 2020, there was a substantial rebound in outpatient clinic care delivered in person (Mehrotra et al., 2020a, 2020b). By October 2020, the percentage of overall telehealth visits continued to slowly decline from a peak in April, but it remained well above the pre-pandemic baseline (Mehrotra et al., 2020c). The data showed significant variation across medical specialties; the proportion of total visits that were delivered via telehealth was lowest among surgical specialties but highest for BH.

Like the broader health care sector, VA rapidly expanded and maintained a high degree of telehealth use for BH care following the onset of the pandemic (Ferguson et al., 2021; VA, 2021). Several researchers have noted that the careful planning, extensive training, and infrastructure support initiatives that facilitated VA's early adoption of telehealth prior to the pandemic were not only instrumental in preparing it to shift to a predominantly virtual health care model during the pandemic, but they also mitigated declines and facilitated continuity of care for patients (Rosen et al., 2021; Zhang, Boden, and Trafton, 2021). VA leaders at the national and local levels used daily and weekly emails and conference calls to support BH providers and disseminated support materials, provided up-to-date guidance on evolving conditions, reiterated available resources to enable virtual care, and shared promising practices (Rosen et al., 2021). Such efforts likely helped VA overcome widely encountered challenges seen elsewhere in the health care sector, such as lack of telehealth familiarity among both patients and providers and inevitable technical challenges.

The pandemic also spurred a rapid expansion of telehealth in the MHS (Larsen, 2020). Innovations, such as leveraging virtual health to extend critical-care resources and treatment at a distance, were used by DHA's Connected Health Branch to facilitate ongoing care delivery through MTFs, according to reports (MHS Communications Office, 2020). The agency further responded to the pandemic with temporary revisions to TRICARE telehealth regulations to expand access to quality care for beneficiaries while minimizing exposure to COVID-19. These provisional changes included giving beneficiaries access to audio-only telephone visits with their providers, a reimbursement qualification for providers who delivered interstate or overseas telehealth, and cost-share and copayment waivers for covered, in-network telehealth services (TRICARE, 2020a). In addition, the TRICARE managed care support contractor Health Net Federal Services, LLC, partnered with telehealth services Doctor On Demand and Telemynd to offer TRICARE West Region beneficiaries increased access to telehealth services (TRICARE, 2020b, 2021), with a focus on patients in remote and rural areas.

Organization of This Report

In this report, we assess the perspectives and experiences of military BH staff regarding their use of telehealth following the onset of the COVID-19 pandemic. These findings informed recommendations to guide the MHS in better integrating telehealth into BH care for service members. We present findings from our interviews with BH staff who delivered or oversaw BH care at MTFs. The semistructured interview protocol asked about their use of telehealth following the onset of the pandemic and factors associated with their use (or nonuse) of telehealth. In Chapter Two, we provide an overview of our methods, including how we selected MTFs and recruited participants, our interview domains, and our analytic approach. In Chapters Three through Seven, we present findings from these interviews. Chapter Eight summarizes our main findings and offers recommendations for integrating telehealth with BH care delivery in the MHS. The interview guide that we used in our interviews with BH staff can be found in the appendix.

CHAPTER TWO

Methods

In this chapter, we describe the methods we used to conduct this study. We begin by describing the process for selecting MTFs and staff at those facilities for our interview sample. We then describe our interview protocol and our qualitative analysis procedures, including our interview coding process. We conclude with a brief description of our interview sample's characteristics. All study methods were approved by RAND's Institutional Review Board, as well as by the DHA Headquarters Human Research Protection Office. In addition, our study procedure received a license from Washington Headquarters Services (DD-HA-2706) as an approved DoD internal information collection procedure.

The onset of the COVID-19 pandemic had a significant impact on this study. We had developed the interview guide prior to the onset of the pandemic and originally intended to conduct in-person interviews at all ten MTFs in spring 2020. Pandemic-related restrictions (e.g., physical distancing, travel limitations) necessitated modifications to the data collection procedures. Our interviews were delayed by several months, and the intended in-person interviews were conducted remotely (i.e., via phone and web-based videoconferencing). The pandemic also influenced the focus of the interviews and this resulting report, with heightened attention and preference given to a rapid analysis of perception of telehealth and experiences using it during the pandemic. These adaptations were implemented not only to account for pandemic-related shift in the originally proposed data collection procedures but also to capture and address the most pressing questions at the time (e.g., how MTF staff were adapting to the rapid increase in telehealth and what lessons their experiences and perspectives could offer for telehealth use in the MHS moving forward). Rather than conduct a quantitative staff survey, we retained the qualitative approach because we expected that the rapid onset of the pandemic and the ensuing challenges to providing behavioral health would lead to a wide variety of responses. Thus, we expected both known unknowns (e.g., the degree to which clinicians employed video telehealth) and unknown unknowns—that is, challenges and adaptive innovations that we would not be able to anticipate *a priori*. Qualitative methods are particularly appropriate in such situations (Rendle et al., 2019).

The revised approach and focus of this study had both strengths and limitations. If we had administered the interview protocol sooner and in person, this report's findings concerning telehealth attitudes, perceptions, and usage rates might have been very different in the absence of a pandemic that caused rapid and major adjustments to the military's delivery of health care.

Interview Sample

We used a tiered stratified sampling approach to maximize the variability of MTFs and staff in our sample. The process and criteria for selecting MTFs and staff members (interviewees), respectively, are described in the following sections.

Military Treatment Facility Selection

In selecting the ten MTFs in our sample, we aimed to maximize variation across four characteristics: service branch, proportion of BH visits with remote service members for the target conditions (PTSD, depression, and SUD), MTF size, and quality of BH care. Table 2.1 provides additional detail on how we defined each characteristic, along with the number of MTFs that were selected in each category. The distribution of selected MTFs leans slightly toward Army MTFs, larger MTFs, and MTFs with higher-quality BH care.

We also aimed to maximize variation in geographic location and whether, to our knowledge, specific telehealth activities occurred at a particular MTF (e.g., whether it was identified as a telehealth hub by a service branch lead). We do not name the selected MTFs in this report; our recommendations are intended for the MHS overall rather than specific MTFs.

Furthermore, although we selected MTFs to maximize variation, the characteristics of these facilities (e.g., quality of BH care) could have changed by the time we conducted our interviews. MTF selection was completed in October 2019 and was based on the data available at that time.[1]

TABLE 2.1

Criteria Informing the Selection of Military Treatment Facilities

Characteristic	Description	Number of MTFs, by Characteristic
Service branch	Army, Navy, Air Force	Army (4) Navy (3) Air Force (3)
MTF size	Total number of direct care visits, divided into three equal groups: • Large: more than 8,000 • Medium: 3,000–8,000 • Small: fewer than 3,000	Large (4) Medium (3) Small (3)
Quality of BH care	Mean quality score derived by averaging quality measure scores assessing care for PTSD, depression, and SUD for patients seen at the MTF, divided into three approximately equal groups of MTFs: • High: above 50% • Average: 40–50% • Low: below 40%	High (5) Average (3) Low (2)
Remote population served	Proportion of BH visits by remote service members for the target conditions: • High: 67–100th percentile; more than 7% remote BH visits • Medium: 34–66th percentile; 2–7% remote BH visits • Low: 0–33rd percentile; less than 2% remote BH visits	High (5) Medium (0) Low (5)

[1] We sampled multiple MTFs across service branches so that our findings would span the diversity of MTF types and clinical contexts. We did not set out *a priori* to make comparisons among service branches.

Interviewee Recruitment

The eligibility criteria for the staff interviews included being (1) a member of the U.S. military (Army, Navy, Air Force, or Marine Corps) in the active component, in the National Guard/reserve (active-duty or active status), or a government/DoD civilian and (2) a provider or administrator who delivered or oversaw care at an MTF for service members who had at least one of the target diagnoses (PTSD, depression, or SUD).[2]

Installation directors of psychological health (or their designee/equivalent, such as the BH department chief/director) were tasked to identify key contacts at the selected MTFs who would work with the research team to coordinate MTF staff interviews. We met with each MTF point of contact, explained the study's goals, and developed a plan for staff recruitment at that MTF. During the discussions, these contacts identified candidate clinics at the MTF (e.g., mental health specialty care, substance use specialty care, primary care) and subsequently provided a list of providers and administrators for us to contact. We invited a mix of provider types to participate in the study to ensure that we captured a wide range of experiences with BH care delivery (including experiences with telehealth). The sample included psychiatrists, psychologists, counselors with a master's in social work (M.S.W.) or other master's degree, substance use counselors, and primary care practitioners.

We aimed to interview approximately eight to ten individuals per MTF, expecting that this number of interviews would provide our analysis with sufficient breadth and depth. Thus, we aimed for a sufficiently comprehensive view of telehealth use at each MTF that we could reliably report on patterns across MTFs. We were able to recruit three to eight respondents per MTF, as some MTFs were smaller than others. We expected (and discovered) considerable variation across MTFs and regions of the United States, as well as variation across clinicians. Thus, we did not aim for complete thematic coverage or saturation across the military health enterprise or across clinicians as a population.

---

[2] Contracted staff were excluded because it was not feasible within the scope of our project to meet the additional regulatory requirements to include them.

Interview Guide

We developed the semistructured interview guide so that it could be used flexibly with a variety of BH provider types in a range of outpatient clinical settings, as well as administrators who oversaw BH care. (The complete guide can be found in the appendix.) Each interview included structured questions to capture military status, service branch, rank, clinical or administrative role (or both), whether the respondent treated service members with each target condition (PTSD, depression, or SUD), location of clinical or administrative activities (e.g., primary care, mental health specialty, SUD specialty), provider type (e.g., psychiatrist, psychologist), and whether the respondent was authorized to prescribe medication.

The interview guide spanned four overarching domains that assessed respondents' perceptions of their approach to treating PTSD, depression, and SUD (when applicable). Although the guide captured a broad set of domains, the decision was made, in conjunction with the study sponsor, to focus this report on staff experiences with and perspectives on the use of telehealth to treat PTSD, depression, and SUD. Table 2.2 lists the domains and associated topics covered in this report.[3] The interview guide included questions designed specifically for providers and administrators; respondents who played both roles could be asked for their perspectives on both providing and overseeing care. Most interview questions included prompts that the interviewer could use to elicit additional responses. For example, regarding experiences with using telehealth, the interviewer could prompt respondents to reflect on specific barriers or facilitators that they encountered while using telehealth to provide treatment. When asking about telehealth options, we defined *telehealth* as "providing treatment via videoconference or telephone or working with patients to use mobile apps to treat or manage symptoms." When discussing the treatment of service members who resided remotely from MTF care, we provided a definition of *remote* as

---

[3] The remaining two domains included in the interview (use of evidence-based care and barriers and facilitators to delivering evidence-based care) are not addressed in this report. The pandemic affected our planned methods and resources, and the focus of this report subsequently shifted to the use of telehealth in the context of the pandemic.

TABLE 2.2
Interview Domains and Associated Topics

Interview Domain	Topics
Telehealth options	• Experience using telehealth to treat PTSD, depression, and SUD (providers)
	• Opinions on telehealth to treat PTSD, depression, and SUD (administrators)
Considerations for remote service members	• Experience treating remote service members and effect on treatment (providers)
	• Considerations when using telehealth with remote service members (providers)
	• Administrative practices used to ensure high-quality care for remote service members (administrators)

residing an hour or more drive away from the MTF. Finally, as we concluded each interview, we invited respondents to provide additional comments.

Data Collection

Interviews were conducted by phone or secure web-based videoconferencing using Microsoft Teams between July and October 2020. Interviews were designed to be 30–45 minutes, but some lasted up to 60 minutes. Incentives were not provided because staff were participating in the interviews during on-duty hours. Staff completed an informed consent process prior to participating in the interview. This consent process clarified that participation was optional and that individual quotations would not include the participant's name or MTF affiliation.

To increase the likelihood that respondents would feel comfortable speaking candidly about their experiences, we did not record the interviews. Instead, one team member listened to the interview while it occurred and typed a near-verbatim account of both interview questions and responses in a Word document. Immediately after the interview, this team member filled gaps and corrected typographical errors. Then, one or more team members who led or assisted with the interview (other than the notetaker) reviewed and edited the document, filling any remaining gaps, redacting any potential identifiers, and adding interviewer notes (in brackets) to provide context for specific statements, when deemed appropriate and helpful for analysis and interpretation. This process allowed us to create a comprehensive, accurate, and organized representation of each interview's content, including some verbatim statements.

Qualitative Data Analysis

Coding Interview Notes

Three research team members were involved in the coding process, which used the team-based qualitative data analytic platform Dedoose, with subsequent data postprocessing in Microsoft Excel. Throughout the coding process, two team members regularly coordinated on coding decisions. The third monitored all coding decisions and led regular meetings with the full research team to review code definitions, code organization, and data aggregation decisions.

Creating *A Priori* Structural Codes

We uploaded all interview notes to Dedoose and employed a combined deductive and inductive approach throughout the coding process. We began with a deductive step. Building on interview domains and the focus of our analysis, we first specified five *a priori* structural codes for interview content. These structural codes formed the basis for how we present our results in Chapters Three through Seven of this report:

- use of telehealth following the onset of the COVID-19 pandemic (Chapter Three)
- organizational factors associated with the use of telehealth (Chapter Four)
- clinical factors affecting the use of telehealth (Chapter Five)
- staff reflections on patient satisfaction and the importance of provider and patient orientation to telehealth (Chapter Six)
- telehealth with service members located remotely from MTF care (Chapter Seven).

Inferring Descriptive and Thematic Subcodes

We followed this deductive step with an inductive analytic step. One team member engaged in an "open-coding" process (Ryan and Bernard, 2000), using interview content to develop subcodes for each structural code. We required these subcodes to have thematic meaning and to be interpretable through a mix of the code name and definition. For example, under the overall structural code "telehealth barriers," one structural code was "MTF staffing/manning inadequate," with the brief definition, "Staffing/manning to support COVID-related changes to telehealth is *currently* inadequate." Code definitions also included specific examples of content for each code; in this case, one of the example quotes for "MTF staffing/manning inadequate" was as follows:

> What has changed [because of the pandemic] is obviously [that] we can do telehealth with them [patients]. Which is not obviously the way therapy is set up, so we're [providers are] having to work every other week from here [alternating between telehealth for "lower-risk" patients one week and in-person care for other patients the next week] due to staffing, everything else that we're down to, so it's pushing out therapy sessions a little further.

This procedure of defining and describing subcodes ensured that the subcodes provided a rich descriptive account of themes observed in the data (organized under the five main structural codes). Because of both the richness and diversity of the interview data—as well as the requirement for each subcode have an independent descriptive thematic meaning—we developed multiple subcodes. For example, the structural code "telehealth barriers" alone contained more than 75 individual subcodes. We emphasized granularity in the initial coding (e.g., distinguishing between audio-only and video telehealth). Similar codes were later merged to enable thematic analysis.

Assigning Interview-Level Variables

To facilitate our demographic analysis and exploration of thematic content across subgroups in the data, we assigned variables to each interview as follows:

- MTF name[4]
- service branch
- military status [military, DoD civilian]
- military rank
- role [clinical/administrative/both/other]
- currently treats service embers with depression [Y/N]
- currently treats service members with PTSD [Y/N]
- currently treats service members with SUD [Y/N]
- location of current clinical or administrative activities [primary care, mental health specialty care, SUD specialty care, integrated mental health/SUD care program, other (specify)]
- provider type [psychiatrist, psychologist, M.S.W./master's-level counselor, SUD counselor, primary care practitioner, other]
- prescriber [Y/N]
- current use of mobile apps [Y/N]
- current use of audio-only telehealth [Y/N]
- current use of video telehealth [Y/N]
- sees remote service members [Y/N]
- mentioned use of telehealth prior to the COVID-19 pandemic[5] [Y/N]
- mentioned use of telehealth with remote service members prior to the COVID-19 pandemic [Y/N]
- mentioned use of telehealth with remote service members during the COVID-19 pandemic [Y/N].

We report summary statistics on these variables in the next section and, in some cases, report thematic prevalence according to these categories throughout this report. Subcodes were included in the analysis if they were endorsed by ten or more respondents or by respondents from three or more

---

[4] Used to produce counts of results by number of MTFs only; results for specific MTFs are not reported.

[5] Some variables (e.g., "Mentioned . . .") were created at the conclusion of coding to provide a denominator for observations. Unlike our structured interview questions, we did not collect these data elements systematically.

MTFs. We included one or more quotations for subcodes endorsed by 20 or more respondents.[6]

Throughout the report, we present counts of respondents who mentioned certain themes. We opted do this for one of two reasons: (1) to illustrate how common or rare certain themes were across our sample and (2) to provide a sense of the relative prevalence of two contrasting or competing themes. It is typical to quantify qualitatively derived themes in research with a sample size of 20 or more. The aim was not to run statistical analyses to estimate point prevalence of specific phenomena or to determine conclusively that one theme was more prevalent than another; rather, we wanted to provide some indication of the prevalence of certain patterns in the data (see Duncan, 2008).

We use standardized terminology to quantify thematic prevalence of responses in which the percentage is tied to the relevant denominator: "few" or "several" for 10 percent or less, "one-quarter" for around 25 percent, "some" for 10–50 percent, "half" for around 50 percent, "most" for more than 50 percent, "three-quarters" for around 75 percent, and "nearly all" for 90 percent and more.

Respondent Characteristics

Key contacts at MTFs provided contact information for 71 BH administrators and providers, ranging from four to nine per MTF. Of these, 53 completed an interview (75-percent raw response rate), and 52 were included in our analyses. One of the completed interviews was excluded because the respondent's role differed significantly from the clinical and administrative roles of other respondents (i.e., the individual was not providing or overseeing treatment). Of those who did not complete an interview, 11 were nonresponders (i.e., they did not respond after three or more attempts), five were ineligible (i.e., they did not provide or oversee BH care for service members

---

[6] In some cases, we included quotations that did not meet this respondent threshold. These cases met one or more of the following conditions: (1) quotes were particularly illustrative or evocative or (2) themes were pertinent to the focal concerns of the study, even if few providers were able to comment on them (e.g., providers who treated remote service members).

at the time of our study, were classified as contractors, or were no longer affiliated with the military), and two declined to participate. The majority of the 52 interviews in our final sample were completed in August and September 2020 (seven interviews conducted in July, 21 in August, 22 in September, and two in October). Table 2.3 presents the employment characteristics of the 52 participants included in our analyses. Participants were primarily DoD government civilians (62 percent) and active-component service members (37 percent). Most (46 percent) had Army affiliations, with less representation from Air Force (31 percent) and Navy (23 percent) MTFs.

TABLE 2.3
Interviewee Characteristics

Characteristics	Participants (N = 52)	
	%	n
Military status		
Active component	36.5	19
DoD government civilian	61.5	32
Reserve	1.9	1
Service branch		
Army	46.2	24
Navy	23.1	12
Air Force	30.8	16
Rank		
E-5–E-9	7.7	4
O-1–O-3	15.4	8
O-4–O-8	13.5	7
N/A	63.5	33
Role		
Clinical only	46.2	24
Both clinical and administrative	51.9	27
Other[a]	1.9	1

Table 2.3—Continued

Characteristics	Participants (*N* = 52)	
	%	*n*
Currently treats service members with[b]		
PTSD	78.8	41
Depression	84.6	44
SUD	71.2	37
Setting of current clinical or administrative activities[b]		
Primary care	5.8	3
Mental health special care	50.0	26
SUD specialty care	30.8	16
Integrated mental health/SUD care program	23.1	12
Other	11.5	6
Provider type		
Psychiatrist	11.5	6
Psychologist	40.4	21
M.S.W./master's-level counselor	25.0	13
SUD counselor	13.5	7
Primary care practitioner	3.8	2
Other	5.8	3
Prescriber		
Yes	19.2	10
No	80.8	42

[a] One participant had an administrative role but did not oversee individuals who provide BH care, and thus did not meet our operational definition of an administrator.

[b] Participants could be included in more than one category.

Fifty-two percent had dual clinical and administrative roles, 46 percent had strictly clinical roles, none had strictly administrative roles, and 2 percent had other responsibilities.

Summary

In this chapter, we provided an overview of our study methods, including recruitment and data collection procedures, along with our data analysis approach. Finally, we described characteristics of those who participated in an interview. In the following chapters, we present findings from our syntheses of these interviews.

CHAPTER THREE

Use of Telehealth Following the Onset of the COVID-19 Pandemic

In this chapter, we summarize staff perceptions on telehealth use at their MTFs, as shared in our interviews, following the onset of the COVID-19 pandemic. We first highlight changes that occurred during the transition from in-person care to audio-only or video telehealth early in the pandemic. We then describe how this initial response evolved as MTFs and staff continued adapting to pandemic-related restrictions on in-person care.

Although our interview protocol did not focus explicitly on pre-pandemic use of telehealth, many staff referenced the pre-pandemic period to contextualize pandemic-related changes in telehealth use. Some indicated that they had used some form of telehealth for care delivery prior to the pandemic ($n = 16$). A portion of these respondents ($n = 8$) mentioned that one or more staff at their MTF were using video telehealth with patients located at other MTFs. Respondents ($n = 10$) from six MTFs mentioned prior experience using telehealth with remote populations (e.g., service members deployed to distant locations outside the continental United States [OCONUS]). At least two MTFs had telehealth managers or other dedicated telehealth staff at the onset of the pandemic. In contrast, several respondents explicitly noted that there were *no* video telehealth treatment options available at their clinic prior to the pandemic, while a few others mentioned that audio-only telehealth was not allowed during that period ($n = 2$). It is important to keep in mind this variation in experience with telehealth among staff when interpreting the findings in this report.

Initial Expansion of Telehealth Use in Response to the COVID-19 Pandemic

Staff described how the first surges of COVID-19 in their respective regions led to abrupt increases in the use of audio-only and video telehealth at their MTFs. Close to half ($n = 21$) of respondents (representing nearly all MTFs) characterized the initial pandemic period as a crisis and said that their MTF experienced a dramatic reduction in care provision, an unsustainable change in the model of care delivery (e.g., treating only the highest-risk patients, replacing visits with short phone calls for safety checks), or the complete cessation of care. According to one Air Force provider, "For a while there, we stopped seeing patients in clinic altogether, unless there was some kind of a situation where we absolutely felt like we had to get someone in the building." Similarly, an Army provider described a period of uncertainty and a disruption in patient care: "So, when COVID first hit, we were coming into the clinic just because I don't think they knew what to do with us, and we were considered to be essential workers. But people [patients] weren't coming in, so that's when we were doing the phone, because people weren't coming in."

Nearly all respondents ($n = 49$) noted a dramatic shift from in-person care to audio-only or video telehealth or a combination of in-person and telehealth modalities during the early pandemic period. One-quarter ($n = 13$) mentioned that this shift occurred quickly—in some cases overnight. As one Army provider/administrator explained it, "We were in clinic, working . . . and literally that afternoon we went home for teleworking and stayed in that posture until [several months later]. So, it was like overnight, go home, call your patients, tell them we're doing this different thing." Another Army provider/administrator said, "I feel like we kind of stumbled into it [telehealth]."

By necessity, this transition involved video telehealth, audio-only telehealth, or modified in-person visits. Most respondents ($n = 32$), representing all MTFs in our study, described significantly increased use of audio-only telehealth, with nearly one-quarter ($n = 9$) saying they used their personal cell phone or home phone to contact patients for audio-only telehealth while working remotely during the pandemic. Sometimes, this was characterized as a stopgap measure (e.g., "They're working on getting me all the tech I need—computers, video camera—but right now I use my personal cell phone, and I have the [Doximity] app").[1] A significant minority also described an increased use of video telehealth ($n = 19$). Less commonly ($n = 2$), providers reported using no audio-only or video telehealth during the pandemic. Several respondents stated that they were "mostly" providing modified in-person care (for example, wearing masks and practicing physical distancing) rather than telehealth ($n = 5$) or providing audio-only or video telehealth by patient request only ($n = 5$).

Early in the pandemic, many providers saw telehealth as a way of providing the minimum necessary care on a temporary basis. Several respondents ($n = 10$) described using telehealth for "check-ins" during this early pandemic period rather than for full-length appointments. They provided multiple reasons for resorting to a check-in–only model. In some cases, this decision was seen as driven by a lack of clear guidance on how to proceed, while in others, it was command-driven and a result of staffing challenges. In the words of one Army provider/administrator,

> Part of it was just kind of being in "oh, shit" mode and being like, "Any care is something." I think that was part of it. I think part of it was this narrative that people were going to fall apart in COVID, so, again, everything became very risk assessment/triage–focused as opposed to actual care. Our experience did not bear that out. [I] can't speak to others, [but] people did not fall apart. People did fine; we did not have to baby them. A lot of people were doing better, actually, not being at work. So, I think that was a missed opportunity—just calling to see if everyone was okay instead of delivering evidence-based treatment still.
>
> Then the other things, I get why, but how do I say this? The culture in COVID was sort of way less checks and balances. And I get why, because everyone was doing the best they could, but that also kind of set a tone, I think, of "You can call your patient and just see how they're feeling about COVID," instead of working on the stuff you've been working on forever. Or, "You can do a 20-minute session instead

---

[1] DHA-approved platforms included Microsoft Skype, Apple FaceTime, and Google Duo beginning in March 2020 (DHA, 2020), followed by the addition of Microsoft Teams in November 2020.

of a 60-minute session." You know what I mean? It just got very sort of loose.

Gradual Return to Delivering In-Person Care

Interviewees also commented on telehealth and care delivery after the initial pandemic response. In this section, we highlight respondents' perspectives on changes they observed as pandemic-related restrictions were lifted and it was possible to see more patients in person, as well as how this related to the ongoing use of telehealth.

Returning to In-Person Care

By the time of our interviews (July–October 2020), most respondents ($n = 30$) across all the MTFs in our sample were increasing in-person visits and returning to something that at least partially resembled their pre-pandemic models of care delivery. Half of respondents ($n = 26$) across all MTFs reported that care delivery at their MTF was "back to normal" or returning to normal. A subset of these staff ($n = 14$) indicated that the increase in telehealth volume initiated during the peak of the pandemic had reverted to previous rates, in part or completely, by the time that we conducted our interviews. Some respondents noted a lack of reliable video telehealth in describing this reversion to previous models of care delivery (e.g., equipment barriers, unreliable technology). Others characterized the return to normal as occurring in the context of a decline in new COVID cases. For example, temporary staffing changes ended or were modified (e.g., nonessential staff returned to the clinic, providers transitioned from telework only to alternating in-person/telework schedules), either as local public health conditions improved or as it "became clear this was going to drag on" and the existing arrangements were no longer sustainable. One respondent cited the large number of enlisted service members at the base as influencing the decision to reopen for in-person care; the service members "liked the idea of getting out of their room [for a BH appointment]" during the garrison lockdown. As one Army provider explained, "At first, people were a little reluctant to come in in person, but now, I don't really have any patients anymore who are not coming in out of concern for their safety."

Current Use of Telehealth

As noted, more than half of respondents told us that the use of audio-only telehealth significantly increased during the early phase of the pandemic, while a little under half said the same about video telehealth. At the time of our interviews, approximately six months into the pandemic, we asked providers (respondents who were delivering care; $n = 51$) about their current use of various telehealth modalities, including audio-only and video telehealth and the integration of mobile apps (Figure 3.1). Nearly all providers (96 percent) reported using at least some audio-only telehealth, while nearly half (41 percent) reported using at least some video telehealth. More than half (59 percent) reported at least some integration of mobile apps into their current BH care delivery. Apps developed by DHA Connected Health (formerly the National Center for Telehealth and Technology) and VA were frequently cited by respondents as apps that they had recommended to patients (DHA, undated c).[2]

As Figure 3.1 highlights, providers reported using video telehealth least often ($n = 21$). Their remarks indicated that video telehealth was difficult to implement. Respondents ($n = 8$) at two of the ten MTFs indicated that their facilities never developed the capability to implement video telehealth during the pandemic, despite a stated interest or willingness to use it on the part of providers ($n = 6$). At five MTFs, respondents ($n = 22$) reported that only one or two providers were using video telehealth at each of their facilities. One prescriber who was using audio-only telehealth during the pandemic stated, "It was all just telephone for us. They never set us up with videoconference." One provider who used both audio-only and video telehealth explained, "I'm talking on speaker right now to my telephone. There's a lot of that. We did video chats, too, but connectivity has been really, really a challenge." In contrast, staff at two MTFs ($n = 14$) reported that at least three providers per MTF were using video telehealth during the pandemic, and respondents from one MTF ($n = 8$) reported that seven providers had been using telehealth. Some had preexisting video telehealth services and

---

[2] Examples included the DHA-offered app Breathe2Relax and the VA apps Mindfulness Coach and PE Coach, with *PE* referring to *prolonged exposure*, a type of therapy provided to patients with PTSD.

FIGURE 3.1

Current Use of Telehealth Modalities at the Time of Our Interviews, July–October 2020, by Modality

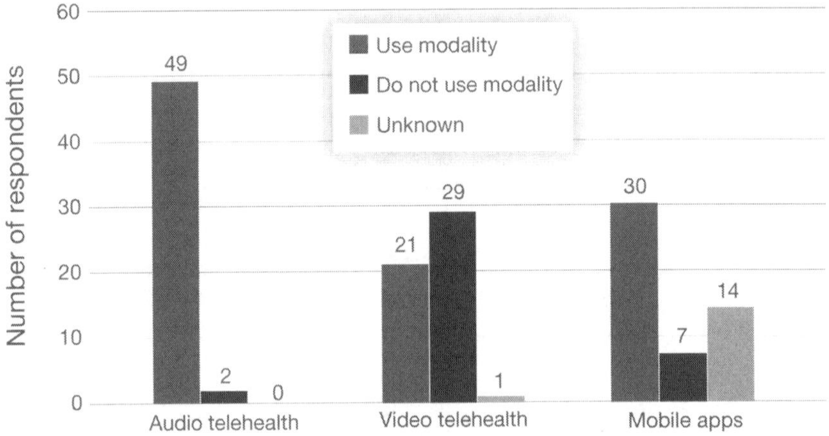

NOTES: Includes providers who delivered BH care (n = 51). "Unknown" indicates that the provider did not mention using the modality.

"COVID just amped up its usage," while others started using video tele-health in response to the pandemic.

As Figure 3.1 reveals, at least some use of audio-only or video telehealth persisted beyond the initial stages of the pandemic at most MTFs. In many cases, it was maintained for only a fraction of patients, or it was used on an as-needed basis. For example, some staff stated that telehealth was used only by request from providers or patients who were at increased risk for serious illness if infected with COVID-19, with patients with stable BH conditions who preferred not to come in, and in other circumstances. In contrast, a notable subset of staff (n = 9) across more than half of the MTFs stated that telehealth was becoming "more normal" as the pandemic continued or that "face-to-face [treatment] is no longer the default." For example, several respondents reported that telehealth was beginning to feel "about the same as normal." Although these remarks were often accompanied by other comments during the interview reflecting the challenges or barriers to continued telehealth use, these respondents indicated that the increased use of telehealth modalities had not changed their overall approach to treatment.

Summary

In this chapter, we characterized the use of telehealth across the ten MTFs in our sample, according to our interviewees. These observations included comparisons with pre-pandemic use of telehealth and updates on the status of telehealth use at the MTFs at the time of our interviews. Nearly all respondents noted a dramatic shift from in-person care to audio-only or video telehealth early in the pandemic or reported that their MTF offered a combination of in-person and telehealth modalities.

At the time of the interviews, nearly all providers (96 percent) reported using at least some audio-only telehealth, while nearly half (41 percent) reported using at least some video telehealth. More than half (59 percent) reported at least some integration of mobile apps into their current BH care delivery approach.

Respondents across MTFs reported differences in the degree to which they increased their use of audio-only and video telehealth. They also described variations in the continued implementation of telehealth, ranging from a return to in-person care delivery to efforts to sustain or expand telehealth use, as well as combinations thereof.

CHAPTER FOUR

Organizational Factors Associated with the Use of Telehealth

In Chapter Three, we described patterns in the use of different telehealth modalities following the onset of the pandemic. We noted that nearly all providers ($n = 49$) were using some form of telehealth to deliver BH care since the onset of the pandemic. In this chapter, we describe staff perspectives on organizational factors related to the effective use of telehealth, including technology, workforce capacity, and policies.

Technological Capacity for Video Telehealth

In this section, we describe respondents' comments on the technology required for video telehealth. Nearly all ($n = 51$) respondents mentioned concerns about having adequate technology to support telehealth. They described inadequate equipment and internet bandwidth, a lack of technical support, problems accessing or using video telehealth platforms, and concerns about data security. We note that we did not document the details of the available technology according to each respondent, so our findings should be interpreted as representative of respondents' perspectives on video telehealth technology in general.

Technological Infrastructure

Technological infrastructure broadly includes required equipment (e.g., computers, webcams), internet connectivity and bandwidth, user-friendly video platforms, data security protocols, and technical support. Nearly all staff ($n = 48$) across all MTFs noted barriers or limitations in technological infrastructure at MTFs, including unmet equipment needs, insufficient internet bandwidth, and a lack of technical support. More than half of respondents, again representing all ten MTFs, mentioned inadequate equipment as a barrier to using telehealth ($n = 28$) and indicated that they did not have access to laptop computers for telework or necessary peripherals for video telehealth, such as cameras. One provider commented on their own equipment compared with that of providers who were delivering video telehealth regularly prior to the pandemic: "At work, I would need the proper equipment. We don't have cameras at all. Our computers are ancient. . . . Our [videoteleconferencing] psychiatrists had good equipment, but ours is quite old." Several respondents also remarked that the equipment they had was not working or that it would malfunction in a way that interfered with their attempts to deliver video telehealth.

Half of respondents ($n = 26$) from all ten MTFs described not having sufficiently reliable internet connectivity or bandwidth. About a third of respondents ($n = 16$) described MTF bandwidth limitations; for example,

> I haven't used it enough yet, but IT people told me the bandwidth for the VPN [virtual private network] is limited by DHA. And there have been multiple complaints, at least among the Navy, about traffic on VPN being so high that it typically would kick people off network or there would be a delayed response.

Similarly, another provider (at an OCONUS location) said,

> I've had that happen, where someone starts to talk about something they're already reluctant to talk about, and the [video] call drops, and I have to ask them to repeat it. And then the call drops again. And, you know, this can go on for ten to 15 minutes until you determine, "Oh, we're just going to talk on the phone." So, we're working on improving it, but it's one of the hesitancies for sure.

Respondents ($n = 12$) from half the MTFs also mentioned challenges related to poor connections at patient locations. One provider recounted, "The barracks are like little stone caves, so not great internet connectivity, so the sessions drop or freeze up." Others pointed out that because of pandemic-related work-from-home orders, video telehealth visits with patients whose spouses were teleworking or who were competing with other family members for bandwidth were often disrupted by poor connections and dropped or frozen calls. Other respondents ($n = 11$) described unreliable connectivity without specifying the root cause. As one provider explained, "Being technology, it's not really reliable. Some things get missed. Sometimes, I'll end [our video telehealth platform] and switch to telephone calls to be sure I'm not missing out on chunks of what they're saying."

In addition to bandwidth and connectivity challenges at the MTFs, some respondents ($n = 14$) described subpar technological infrastructure more generally. For example, one provider whose MTF had not yet implemented video telehealth stated, "We're a very large bureaucracy, and we tend to use yesterday's technology tomorrow." Others ($n = 24$) described an overall lack of reliability of video telehealth, in particular, without identifying specific barriers. Finally, several respondents ($n = 7$) across half of MTFs voiced concerns about the lack of technical support at their MTF, with one respondent suggesting that "there seemed to be virtually no technical support" for video telehealth during the pandemic.

Telehealth Platforms and Data Security

Most respondents ($n = 39$) expressed frustrations related to telehealth platforms, interoperability, and data security. And most of them ($n = 35$) reported difficulty accessing or using platforms for video telehealth while working from home or in the office during the pandemic. About a third of providers ($n = 18$) mentioned that DHA-approved platforms (e.g., Cisco Meeting, Adobe Connect) were unreliable or not user-friendly. Meanwhile, 11 providers (from nearly all MTFs) expressed uncertainty about which platforms were approved, noting that guidance seemed to change frequently. Some providers stated that, after learning to use what they thought was an approved platform for video telehealth, they believed the policy changed and that the platform was no longer allowed. Relatedly, several providers ($n = 3$) mentioned that there were platforms that they believed were approved by DHA but not permitted by their local MTF or vice versa. Respondents also reported issues with firewalls and interoperability ($n = 5$) or stated that a complete lack of access to a video telehealth platform was preventing them from using video telehealth ($n = 8$). For example, one provider explained,

> We sound like we are abandoning our patients here, but, I mean, we contacted them weekly—if not bimonthly—there. And basically, you know, it was 30 minutes to an hour [of an audio-only session]. Our [IT] folks did push out Microsoft Teams on our computers here, but they haven't really given us access, and a lot of us don't have cameras. We have desk[top] computers here, so it's not like we have cameras where we could participate here. I even tried. . . . So, yeah, Zoom meetings, Microsoft Teams, didn't work for us here. Most of us did our telehealth through the phone.

Providers also said they wished that they could use popular platforms available to civilian providers during the pandemic. Eleven respondents commented specifically that Zoom was not allowed, and five of them expressed frustration at not being permitted to use it. One explained,

> This day and age we're dealing with 18-year-olds and up to 60s, and they have different apps. Zoom, FaceTime. If I say only [Adobe Connect], I will lose half of them because they either don't like it, don't want it, phone is not compatible with it. So, I don't see why we can't use whatever they prefer.

More than one-quarter of respondents ($n = 19$) mentioned provider or patient concerns about data security and privacy as a barrier to using video telehealth effectively. Some stated that they believed patients preferred audio-only telehealth because of these privacy concerns, even with HIPAA- and DHA-approved platforms, such as Cisco or Adobe Connect. Providers themselves did not express security concerns about these platforms. However, when certain HIPAA provisions were relaxed during the pandemic and alternative platforms were offered at some MTFs (e.g., Skype, FaceTime), some providers were concerned about data security. According to one provider, such platforms "can't necessarily promise a secure connection."

Technology Solutions and Workarounds

Few respondents mentioned solutions to these types of technology challenges. Several ($n = 5$) said that their MTF used strategies to increase internet connectivity during the pandemic, such as purchasing additional bandwidth ($n = 2$) or switching internet providers ($n = 2$). Meanwhile, one person stated that their clinic had purchased an "enhancement platform" for better Cisco Meeting connectivity and that their MTF had sent providers home to telework to free up on-site bandwidth.

Four respondents at one MTF described using an app designed in house for delivering video telehealth. The app offered patients and providers a secure means of connecting for video telehealth appointments, and it could be used from a smartphone, laptop, or desktop computer. Two respondents at this same MTF also mentioned using DoD SAFE (Secure Access File Exchange) to have patients sign treatment-related documents. Finally, respondents ($n = 4$) at four MTFs described building process templates in the electronic health record or practice management system for scheduling and coding for telehealth.

In terms of solutions to telehealth technology challenges, one staff member suggested that DHA create "a DHA app" for delivering video telehealth. Another suggested that DHA acquire an electronic medical record with an embedded video telehealth capability.

Administrative Tasks, Symptom Tracking, and the Behavioral Health Workforce

In this section, we summarize staff perceptions related to the relationship between telehealth and conducting patient care–related administrative tasks and the adequacy of the BH workforce.

Administrative and Logistical Challenges

Most staff ($n = 31$) across all MTFs described administrative barriers to implementing telehealth. These included logistical barriers ($n = 20$), such as scheduling appointments and documenting sessions while providers were teleworking, and monitoring symptoms ($n = 11$). Nearly one-quarter of respondents (n = 16) described logistical challenges to video telehealth, while fewer (n = 5) encountered logistical challenges with audio-only telehealth. Additional challenges included needing to complete paperwork or obtain patient signatures prior to the first telehealth visit (n = 5) and sharing and collecting therapy-related handouts and "homework" (i.e., between-session activities to practice skills introduced in the session; n = 6).

Symptom Tracking via the Behavioral Health Data Portal

Nearly one-quarter of respondents (n = 11) reported challenges with symptom tracking. Prior to the pandemic, BH treatment included routine symptom assessments for PTSD, depression, and anxiety (DHA Procedural Instruction 6490.02, 2018). MHS providers used a web-based application, the Behavioral Health Data Portal (BHDP), to collect these data from patients through waiting room kiosks or tablets (DoD, 2016). The BHDP generates graphs of symptom changes over time. During the pandemic, concerns about COVID transmission prohibited the use of BHDP via kiosks or shared tablets, which made it difficult for providers to track patient symptoms. Even those who later developed strategies for collecting this information orally or in writing found it challenging to track patient outcomes without the help of the portal's automatic reminders and graphs to show symptom changes.

Notably, although lack of patient access to BHDP was a challenge for some providers, several (n = 8) reported finding novel adaptations. For example, two providers used email to collect BHDP symptom measures from patients, with one explaining that they created an Excel file with each measure in a separate tab for patients to complete and return via email prior to their audio-only telehealth visit. In addition, several providers (n = 5) told us they developed a practice of administering BHDP symptom measures orally during audio-only or video telehealth visits. One respondent suggested that, in the future, it would be helpful if the MHS "could take the BHDP to an app."

Behavioral Health Workforce

About half of all staff (n = 28) reported that they believed existing workforce challenges could hamper telehealth growth and sustainment, including inadequate staffing ($n = 21$), attrition ($n = 15$), and burnout ($n = 10$) among providers. About a quarter of respondents ($n = 14$) reported a lack of adequate clinical staff to meet the demand for telehealth appointments, and a smaller number ($n = 10$) described inadequate staffing as a possible barrier to using telehealth in the future. For example, one provider explained that providers at their MTF would use audio-only telehealth during the pandemic "in some arenas" but that this "depends on manning," or the number of MTF providers. Similarly, a respondent at an OCONUS location explained,

> A while back when I first got here, we had way more staff than we do now. And we were doing a lot more VTC [videoteleconferencing]. . . . So, I have done that. We had the bandwidth to do it then. Then, as we started losing staff, and we started to tighten up, and we had to stop doing telehealth to all of these outlying places. Which is a huge problem out here . . . because you just can't go into town and find a therapist. So, it's been more of an access problem. But we have started a bit of it back up again. But not much. But it's an access issue more than anything.

Remarks about attrition were more varied. Staff ($n = 4$) at three MTFs reported that delays in filling vacant provider positions were negatively influencing their ability to use telehealth during the pandemic, and nearly one-quarter of respondents ($n = 11$) described provider staffing shortages as a potential threat to use of telehealth in the future. Others mentioned MTF leadership discontinuity ($n = 2$) or a need to train newly hired providers ($n = 2$) as associated challenges.

Finally, providers ($n = 10$) cited burnout as a potential barrier to the sustained use of telehealth. Several described provider caseloads as being "too high" or work as being "pretty fast-paced" or "a tough gig," leaving little bandwidth for providers to successfully transition to video telehealth. Concomitantly, four providers indicated that they thought telehealth made their work less efficient than before.

In contrast, several respondents ($n = 6$) noted that they believed telehealth alleviated provider staffing issues, while five respondents across four MTFs noted that the use of telehealth increased efficiency. Several also observed that no-shows were less frequent via telehealth than in person and that the opportunity to work from the home allowed for greater availability and reduced occupational stress. One provider explained that telehealth allowed providers who were exposed to COVID-19 to continue safely seeing their patients, thereby helping to avoid staffing issues that would have resulted if that provider had to transfer all or part of their caseload while quarantining.

Policy Guidance and Leadership Support

In this section, we describe staff perspectives on the need for telehealth-related policy guidance and support from MTF and DHA leadership.

Nearly one-quarter of respondents ($n = 23$) across eight MTFs described inconsistent messages from MTF leadership, bureaucratic "red tape," concerns about approaches to monitoring quality or productivity, or a general lack of MTF support as barriers to the implementation of telehealth efforts. Most of these providers shared positive perceptions of telehealth but also voiced displeasure about how it was being implemented at their MTF (e.g., in ways that disincentivized its use). For example, one provider believed that the relative value units (RVUs, the standardized metric used by the MHS to measure provider productivity) differed for telehealth versus in-person visits:

> Just in the practice sector, the value—the RVUs, the value metrics—need to be the same for telehealth as it is for a face-to-face visit. It never has been, and there were moves in that direction during the lockdown time. From what I understand, the way we code for telehealth doesn't generate RVUs [the same way] as in-person. And we do the same exact work, everything is exactly the same, so I'm not sure why it's not as valuable when it's done as telehealth versus in-person. They even told us that. During lockdown, they said, "We know we'll have to take a hit in productivity during lockdown. Put safety first." But we figured out how to do the math again, and [they started talking about it again, and] they started bringing us back into the hospital. I'm doing the same amount of work and it's the same complexity level, then it ought to be the same as if it's done by telemedicine versus face to face.

Respondents also described unhelpful responses to requests for resources or technical support, with four stating that their MTF did not provide necessary training for providers on the use of telehealth.

Nearly one-quarter of respondents ($n = 22$) across seven MTFs described a lack of support or unclear guidance from DHA on telehealth implementation. Respondents also said that DHA policy guidance (including on approved telehealth platforms) was constantly shifting or described cases in which DHA guidance conflicted with local or regional MTF guidance on telehealth. One respondent explained, "DHA and I think [U.S. Army Medical Command] has said, 'You can use FaceTime and Google Duo, but locally we have not been given the okay to do that.' I think Skype is another one that is authorized but we're not allowed to use."

Summary

In this chapter, we highlighted some organizational barriers to the use of telehealth across the ten MTFs in our sample as reported by our interviewees. Nearly all respondents across all MTFs expressed concerns about having adequate technology to support telehealth. Staff also voiced concerns about inadequate equipment and internet bandwidth, lack of technical support, lack of access to video telehealth platforms, and data security.

Most staff across the MTFs in our sample described administrative and logistical barriers to implementing telehealth, such as scheduling appointments while teleworking, documenting sessions, exchanging paperwork, and symptom monitoring. About half described workforce-related barriers to telehealth growth and sustainment, including inadequate staffing, attrition, and burnout. Finally, staff from most MTFs expressed frustration with bureaucratic barriers, unclear guidance, or a perceived lack of support for telehealth at the DHA or MTF level.

CHAPTER FIVE

Clinical Factors Affecting the Use of Telehealth

In this chapter, we present staff perspectives on the appropriateness and utility of telehealth for different types of patients and in different clinical circumstances, including

- high-risk or high-severity patients
- treatment for PTSD or SUD
- group therapy
- initiating treatment with new patients
- unique patient issues and individual differences.

General Attitudes Toward Using Telehealth for Behavioral Health Care

Most respondents (n = 33) across nearly all MTFs stated that increased telehealth use was necessary during the pandemic because of the need to minimize the risk of COVID-19 transmission. Staff also shared their attitudes toward specific modalities: audio-only telehealth, video telehealth, and mobile apps. As noted in Chapter Three, nearly all respondents were using audio-only telehealth at the time of our interviews (n = 49). However, only about one-quarter of these providers (n = 13) expressed an openness to continuing to use audio-only telehealth, and nearly all (n = 12) of those who were open to continued audio-only telehealth also expressed one or more concerns about using it in certain circumstances (e.g., intake appointments, group treatment).

Trends in provider openness to video telehealth were more favorable, yet fewer respondents reported current use of this modality. Among providers who reported using video telehealth at the time of our interviews ($n = 21$), nearly three-quarters ($n = 15$) expressed an openness to continuing to use it in the future. Among clinicians who were not yet using video telehealth ($n = 30$), more than three-quarters expressed at least some degree of openness to using it in the future ($n = 24$). Thus, roughly three-quarters of all respondents expressed at least some degree of openness to video telehealth ($n = 39$). However, only a minority ($n = 9$) expressed enthusiasm for future or continued use of video telehealth without also noting concerns; most respondents ($n = 31$) mentioned potential drawbacks. For example, staff voiced concerns about using video telehealth to manage patient risk (e.g., suicidal ideation), to provide care for particular diagnoses (e.g., SUD, PTSD), and to initiate care with new patients (e.g., establishing rapport).

Finally, when asked about mobile health apps, some staff ($n = 19$) expressed positive attitudes. Several were already using apps to augment in-person or virtual treatment ($n = 14$). These providers actively encouraged patients to use apps developed by DHA Connected Health (e.g., Breath2Relax) and VA (e.g., Mindfulness Coach, PE Coach) to track symptoms, complete homework, receive medication reminders, or practice new skills between sessions. As one provider explained, "I'm not typically substituting face-to-face or other formal video care treatment with the apps, but I augment most—with most of my patients—just [with] good stress management and relaxation and other skills." Others reported that they recommended apps to patients during intake visits or as needed without fully integrating app use into their clinical practice. According to one respondent, "Yes, so we have a handout from the DoD and they're not DoD apps but they're somewhat screened, so I do hand that out. I have a bunch of them in my office, and I give them to patients who are open to that."

A small number of respondents ($n = 4$) across four MTFs expressed concern about a perceived lack of evidence for audio-only and video telehealth. One provider/administrator said, "I'm not sure everyone would agree with me that it [telehealth] is an equivalent form of care, but I think that most people would agree that it is a good way to provide care in most circumstances." Another provider/administrator observed, "If telehealth was so great and we knew this already, we should have been doing this before."

Another remarked that more research is needed to compare patient outcomes for in-person care versus telehealth: "I think people would have more confidence if there were actually a study or research-based evidence that it is effective or at least close."

Some respondents (*n* = 9) told us they viewed telehealth as "the future" of BH care delivery. One respondent said, "I personally think telehealth is a good thing and the way forward." Another noted that COVID was "going to be a big game-changer for behavioral health in the future, for better or worse." Notably, of the nine respondents who saw telehealth as the future of BH care, fewer than half had used video telehealth during the pandemic.

Nearly all respondents (*n* = 50 across all ten MTFs) remarked in some way about clinical and treatment-related factors influencing the appropriateness of telehealth. Thus, although several staff reported being open to or having positive perceptions of various telehealth modalities, our interviewees frequently expressed concerns about using telehealth across a variety of clinical situations. In the sections that follow, we describe five major areas of concern.

High-Risk or High-Severity Patients

The first clinical theme that emerged when this topic came up related to the use of telehealth with high-risk patients or patients with high symptom severity. Most respondents commented in some way about the appropriateness of telehealth to treat patients with high symptom severity (*n* = 33). Specifically, they mentioned concerns about patients who were on a designated "high-interest list," for whom safety issues were present, who expressed suicidal ideation, who were recently hospitalized, or who were discharged from other inpatient settings, such as intensive outpatient programs. Respondents across all ten MTFs expressed concern about the use of telehealth with this population (*n* = 28), while a smaller number expressed enthusiasm (*n* = 2) or a mix of concern and enthusiasm (*n* = 3).

Concerns were specifically raised about use of both audio-only and video telehealth with these patients, although slightly more respondents raised concerns about audio-only telehealth (*n* = 23) than video telehealth (*n* = 17). Comments pertaining to audio-only telehealth, in particular, often reflected providers' unease at not being able to assess nonverbal cues that might indicate elevated symptoms, particularly if a patient was reluctant to report their symptoms. One psychiatrist said, "The ones [patients] with higher acuity seeing a social worker every week, a psychologist every week, and me every two weeks—they are not appropriate for that [audio-only telehealth]. . . . If you're a cutter, recently hospitalized, in trouble at work, then yeah, you need to come see me." Most providers and administrators stated that high-risk or high-acuity patients or those with suicidal ideation were typically seen in person during the pandemic ($n = 25$). Several providers who used audio-only telehealth said that they would switch to in-person sessions during the course of therapy if their patient began to exhibit elevated distress, regardless of whether it was the result of an existing or new problem ($n = 6$).

Meanwhile, respondents across most MTFs mentioned that telehealth was appropriate to treat mild to moderate BH conditions ($n = 14$). They explicitly acknowledged being comfortable with conducting sessions via audio-only ($n = 12$) or video ($n = 8$) telehealth for a range of conditions, such as depression, SUDs, anxiety disorders, adjustment disorder, relationship issues, and even PTSD, provided that patients exhibited stable and lower-acuity symptoms. As one provider put it,

> What I can say is that the term used quite often is *the new normal*, but the new normal in treatment—from what I've seen and told patients to expect, rather than routinely telling people, more so with depression and substance use disorders—face-to-face is no longer the default for every encounter. If someone is stable and making measurable progress and would benefit from telehealth, then we gravitate toward telehealth to see what is going on and see what is needed from there. Of course, this is after an evaluation.

Treatment for PTSD and Substance Use Disorders

The second major clinical theme that emerged related to concerns about the use of telehealth to treat PTSD and SUD. Although treatment for depression was discussed by several respondents, these remarks did not meet our threshold for reporting (unless there were concerns about suicidality or other high-risk patient characteristics, which were more dominant themes).

Use of Telehealth for PTSD

Of the 42 providers who reported treating PTSD, 17 commented about the appropriateness of telehealth for PTSD treatment. Most ($n = 14$) expressed concerns, while a few ($n = 3$) expressed a combination of concern and enthusiasm. Providers were about as likely to express concern or reluctance about treating PTSD via audio-only telehealth ($n = 13$) as via video telehealth ($n = 10$). Most respondents expressing concern about audio-only telehealth indicated that it was not conducive to evidence-based psychotherapies for PTSD (such as prolonged exposure, cognitive processing therapy, or eye movement desensitization reprocessing), in part because the provider was not able to see whether a patient was decompensating, engaging in nonverbal avoidance behaviors, or demonstrating visual cues of dissociation during the treatment session. Although some providers refused to deliver any PTSD treatment via audio-only telehealth, others opted to avoid exposure elements in favor of focusing more on the cognitive-behavioral aspects of treatment. Still others switched to purely supportive therapy with their patients during the pandemic.

Staff voiced similar concerns regarding video telehealth for PTSD treatment. In addition, multiple providers described experiences in which connectivity issues led to a video call failing multiple times during imaginal exposure exercises, leading both provider and patient to agree not to conduct future sessions by video. As one provider explained,

> I think there has to be better platforms. If you can guarantee me that I'm not going to going to lose connectivity 15 minutes into the session, or you won't be pixelated, or the sound won't go out, or whatever the case may be, I would be comfortable doing more trauma work, because I wouldn't be concerned that then the patient would be out there and in a bad place [after losing the connection].

Use of Telehealth for Substance Use Disorders

Twelve respondents discussed the appropriateness of telehealth for the treatment of SUDs. Most were treating patients with these conditions, and all were providers or dual providers/administrators. Several providers expressed concern ($n = 5$), while others expressed a mix of concern and enthusiasm ($n = 4$) or expressed enthusiasm only ($n = 3$).

Concerns usually centered around treating high-risk SUD patients or patients with severe SUD symptoms. Some providers believed that the pandemic affected patients in various ways that made treatment more challenging (e.g., by making group support infeasible, introducing new stressors at home, or lifting requirements for random drug testing). Some felt that rates of relapse had increased during the pandemic.

Providers expressed concern about treating SUD via audio-only telehealth ($n = 9$) and video telehealth ($n = 4$). Among those using audio-only telehealth, some providers indicated that this modality made it impossible to assess for certain visual signs of withdrawal, and one provider commented that it may be more difficult to assess for relapse while using audio-only telehealth. According to one Army provider, "The worrisome stuff is the logistics of it. Being able to fully evaluate nonverbal stuff with clients . . . especially SUD clients—to be able to pick up on whether the patient is intoxicated, experiencing delirium, or having the shakes." Respondents also remarked that some patients may be more difficult to engage in treatment using audio-only telehealth.

Respondents who expressed concern about treating SUDs via video telehealth ($n = 4$) shared many of the same sentiments. Providers remarked that some aspects of a mental status exam are challenging to complete even via video telehealth, making it difficult to assess for intoxication and symptoms of delirium tremens, such as shaking or sweating. One SUD provider who was not using any telehealth at the time of our interview commented that they would potentially be comfortable using video telehealth with stable SUD patients but not with patients who are more acute or who are not stable in their abstinence:

> How do I view it? I would say I have mixed feelings. . . . I think primary provision of services to people with moderate to severe diagnosis needs to be continuing face to face. Telehealth—the actual treatment

for this population—needs to have some face-to-face component for it, with this population. Somebody with a mild diagnosis [of alcohol use disorder], I'm a little flexible there because their goal is flexible use. Again, [we would] still need to call those in for random urinalysis to keep them honest, but typically what we do is an EtG, Ethyl Glucuronide [test].

Seven providers specifically mentioned that audio-only telehealth could be used to treat stable SUD patients who were receiving maintenance medication therapy or psychotherapy, and four of these providers also endorsed video telehealth for the same purposes. Of note, only one-third (n = 12) of the providers who were treating service members with SUDs (n = 37) offered comments about the appropriateness of telehealth to treat these conditions.

Group Therapy

The third clinical theme that emerged was related to group therapy. Due to pandemic-related precautions and the need for physical distancing, many MTFs suspended group treatment even if individual sessions or other aspects of care continued to be offered in person. Specifically, at the time of our interviews, respondents frequently reported that group therapy had been temporarily discontinued at their MTF or that group sessions had been converted to individual sessions (n = 14). An additional six respondents mentioned that there were significantly fewer options for group treatment during the pandemic. Although we did not specifically query staff about whether group treatment was currently being offered, only one respondent indicated that group treatment had continued uninterrupted.

Thirteen respondents commented on the appropriateness of telehealth for group therapy. Traditional in-person group therapy is typically conducted with eight to ten patients, requiring a large room at the facility. Several respondents expressed concern or hesitation about using telehealth for this purpose (n = 9), one expressed both concern and enthusiasm, and three shared only positive remarks. Among the respondents who expressed concerns about telehealth for group therapy, many believed that group therapy could not be conducted over the phone but did not provide a reason for this perspective (n = 10). Concerns about using video telehealth for group facilitation were less frequent ($n = 4$) and mainly reflected respondents' experiences using video telehealth to treat patients individually (e.g., problems with bandwidth, hypothetical concerns about patients not being motivated or engaged, suggestions that the group dynamic might be difficult to emulate virtually).

Initiating Treatment with New Patients

The fourth clinical theme captured concerns about initiating treatment with new patients. Respondents across nearly all MTFs expressed concern about using telehealth to conduct intake assessments or suggested that telehealth should be used with established patients only ($n = 17$). Several ($n = 14$) explained that audio-only telehealth would make it difficult to establish rapport and trust with new patients, to socialize them to the therapy process, and to gain an understanding of their mannerisms and idiosyncrasies. One provider recounted the following experience:

> I was thinking about specifically related to intake. I was assigned a new patient, and this was when we were on phone only—or I was phone-only at home. The intake was especially difficult, having never met the person, not being able to see them, having no idea how to do a history with them. People who I had been seeing before I was still able to pick up on the phone if they were pausing more than normal, how is their voice tone and inflection, but with the new patient I had no history or information: Is this normal, what's going on with the patient? I basically said I'm not going to do any more intakes on the phone. They can see someone else or wait for some exception for me to just have them come into the office because I just really felt strongly that it was not good. And it significantly impacted rapport building and just a really rocky way to start.

Several of the respondents who preferred to conduct intakes in person also said that the process would help them decide whether a patient was a candidate for future telehealth sessions.

Considering Patients' Individual Differences

The fifth and final theme regarding the clinical appropriateness of telehealth spanned a variety of concerns about individual patient characteristics. Twelve respondents suggested that certain types of patients might not respond well to telehealth, although six of these respondents also said that telehealth could be used effectively to treat some or most of their patients.

Providers who expressed concerns about using audio-only telehealth with selected patients ($n = 11$) said that some patients struggled with the phone as a medium for therapy or medication management. One Army provider described this as "an issue of object permanence," explaining that, for some patients, "it's hard for them to hold onto me, the therapy, without seeing me." Other providers cited a patient's "openness" to treatment or "insight" into problems as important variables, explaining that some patients seemed less likely to engage over the phone. At least one provider observed that it appeared even more challenging to create a natural and conversational atmosphere during phone sessions with male patients:

> I would say 75 percent of my patients are males. They're not great on the phone. They're just like, "No, ma'am. Yes, ma'am. Yes. No. Thank you." And I can do a quote—45-minute appointment—in five minutes. There is no time for that give-and-take conversation and letting things come out naturally. It tends to be just direct questioning.

Comparatively fewer providers expressed concerns about using video telehealth with certain patients ($n = 7$ across seven MTFs). In describing the situations in which they would be reluctant to use video telehealth, providers commented that certain patients seemed less comfortable or less engaged. Shyness or introversion were suggested as possible reasons the patient might be uncomfortable appearing on camera. One provider commented on the fact that certain serious BH conditions or symptoms could make video telehealth particularly challenging for patients (e.g., paranoia, delusions, cognitive disturbance).

Summary

This chapter explored the clinical factors that influenced respondents' perspectives on telehealth. Roughly three-quarters expressed at least some degree of openness to continued or future use of video telehealth, while only about a quarter expressed openness to continuing to use audio-only telehealth. At least one-third were open to integrating mobile apps.

About half of respondents expressed concerns about using telehealth to treat high-risk patients or those with high symptom severity. Nearly one-third expressed at least some concern regarding telehealth for PTSD, and nearly one-fifth reported similar opinions when it came to SUD treatment. However, most providers who expressed concern about using telehealth for SUDs also suggested that it could be used appropriately with patients whose conditions are stable. Furthermore, about one-quarter of all respondents suggested that telehealth could be used appropriately to treat mild to moderate BH conditions.

About one-quarter of respondents mentioned that group therapy sessions had stopped at their MTF since the onset of the pandemic, and about one-fifth expressed concerns about using of telehealth to deliver group therapy. Across the MTFs in our sample, about one-third of respondents expressed concerns about using telehealth to conduct intake assessments or suggested that telehealth should be used with established patients only.

CHAPTER SIX

Staff Reflections on Patient Satisfaction and the Importance of Provider and Patient Orientation to Telehealth

In this chapter, we first describe how BH staff at MTFs perceived patient preferences regarding telehealth. Then, we highlight how providers learned to use telehealth on the job (including socializing patients to these modalities).

Staff Perceptions of Patient Preferences Regarding Telehealth

Staff offered their views regarding patient perspectives and preferences, including how telehealth may have helped sustain or improve patients' access to care. Just over half of staff ($n = 27$) reported that they believed patients liked telehealth. Ten of these respondents stated that they believed patients liked telehealth because it increased access to BH care during the pandemic by making it more convenient. Staff noted that telehealth saved driving time, allowed patients to get care if they did not have a vehicle or had lost their driving privileges, and gave them the option of obtaining medication refills over the phone rather than needing to come in (thus reducing wait times in the clinic and time away from work). Providers also talked about being able to reach patients in geographically separated units who might have otherwise encountered too many challenges to seek treatment at an MTF. One provider/administrator who used audio-only and video tele-health explained,

> I just think it's been such a blessing to improve, well really to reduce attrition and improve continuity of care. In our facility like I'm sure many, we have geographically isolated units. We have . . . people . . . who are super-isolated and spend a lot of time isolated in rooms with no windows, miles away from us with officers breathing down their neck, and it's not hard to understand why they might be reluctant to come into our brick-and-mortar clinic. For the ones who do love it [telehealth], they can sit in their car . . . [participate in a session while] on a walk, or sit at home in sweatpants, and God forbid they do have COVID, they can process that. Sessions are a bit shorter, and probably we have fewer screeners with [the] telehealth process, but we've had a considerable drop in attrition. We heard previously that "it was just too hard to come in," but with telehealth, they're telling me, "This is the best thing ever. I really need to talk to you today, but I can't come in, so let's do that."

Providers also discussed how telehealth could help ameliorate patient concerns about mental health stigma. As one provider/administrator who used audio-only and video telehealth during the pandemic explained, some patients preferred telehealth (over in-person care) because it is "anony-mous" and allowed them access to BH care without having to "walk in the building."

Many respondents (n = 23) described instances in which patients expressed a preference for a specific visit modality (i.e., audio-only tele-health, video telehealth, or in-person). Ten providers observed that patients generally liked audio-only telehealth, with several (n = 7) suggesting that patients prefer it to in-person care, and four stated that some patients pre-ferred audio-only over video telehealth. Providers suggested that this was due to the lower logistical burden, greater anonymity, and less social anxiety involved with audio-only telehealth.

In contrast, nearly one-third of respondents (n = 16) said that some of their patients disliked telehealth or preferred in-person care. Although respondents indicated that patients had adapted to telehealth during the pandemic, they noted that some wanted to return to the clinic for sessions as soon as possible. Staff said that these were often patients who had trouble finding a private space at home. A few others said that they had patients who did not trust that video or audio-only transmission of information was private or noted that some patients had a hard time working with the technology.

Familiarizing Providers and Patients to Telehealth

Staff described a "learning curve" for telehealth. They also commented on the importance of preparing patients for their telehealth visits.

Provider Familiarity with Telehealth

A third of staff (n = 18) described navigating a learning curve in which they gradually became more comfortable as they oriented themselves to telehealth modalities. Provider comments included, "I learned from doing," "Necessity will make a lot of things happen," "There is a steep learning curve," and "This is all a learning process." As one administrator observed,

> Initially, there were some grumblings about having to move in this direction, but the vast majority [of providers] have really gotten on board and have been invested in learning the various systems and platforms. Even venturing out into this new one, Doximity,[1] they've found that to be really useful. So, I would say the providers have really accepted it and even, we've kind of collectively grown together.

Several others observed a link between their comfort level with delivering an evidence-based psychotherapy face to face and their comfort level delivering that therapy via telehealth. According to one respondent, "The more comfortable the provider is with the evidence-based practice, the more likely they are to be innovative with the technology." Although comments about the need for specific training in telehealth did not come up frequently

---

[1] DHA-approved platforms included Microsoft Skype, Apple FaceTime, and Google Duo beginning March 2020 (DHA, 2020), followed by the addition of Microsoft Teams in November 2020.

in our interviews, four respondents stated that their MTF did not provide necessary training for providers on the use of telehealth.

Preparing Patients for Telehealth

More than one-third of respondents (n = 23) from most MTFs also referenced a patient "learning curve." As one administrator/provider explained, "There is a learning curve for patients: Will you treat this as a real session even though you're not here? A lot of people just want to do a quick conversation and we're like, settle down, we're going to sit down for 45 or 60 minutes of whatever for therapy, so orienting patients to that [is important] as well." More than half of these providers described situations in which they felt like the patient was not taking the telehealth appointment seriously at first. Examples included patients appearing to forget about appointments, not being in a private space, multitasking during the appointment, or treating the session like a regular phone call with a friend. One clinician made the following comments when describing this dynamic:

> We've had patients using the bathroom while on [our video telehealth platform]. People driving, in bed, rolling out of bed. It just doesn't maybe feel like a real appointment to them, so there has been repeated education on virtual etiquette: This is a real appointment, treat it like any other visit, don't be eating or using the bathroom or those types of things. That has been something that has changed, having to do that education.

In discussing the issue, staff noted that telehealth sessions typically ran more smoothly after they provided instruction and socialized patients to the new modalities. Patients thus grew more accustomed to telehealth sessions over time. One provider created their own version of instructions for video telehealth for patients, explaining, "I made a cheat sheet that wasn't three to four pages [like the standard materials provided by the government], and I could email or text it [to patients]." This respondent observed that the recommended practice of emailing long-form instructions to patients was ineffective, which is what prompted this person "to be versatile about how we're getting the information to them [patients]."

Summary

As part of our interviews, providers reported on their perspectives on patient reception to telehealth. Just over half of staff reported that they believed patients liked telehealth, largely citing the increased convenience associated with telehealth. Staff noted that telehealth addressed transportation barriers and saved patients time away from duties, which are conveniences that would likely still be perceived as beneficial even after the pandemic. In contrast, nearly one-third of providers said some of their patients disliked telehealth or preferred in-person care.

A third of staff described navigating a learning curve in which they gradually became more comfortable with telehealth modalities. A similar proportion of respondents from most MTFs also referenced a patient learning curve, noting that patients needed to be prepared if telehealth visits were going to be as effective as in-person visits.

CHAPTER SEVEN

Telehealth with Service Members Located Remotely from MTF Care

Service members who reside remotely from an MTF experience challenges accessing high-quality BH care. Our prior research showed that remote service members are much more likely to receive their BH care from private-sector providers (i.e., TRICARE-contracted providers in the community) as opposed to MTFs (Hepner et al., 2021). Still, we asked staff for their perspectives on providing BH care to *remote* service members, defined during our interviews as those located at a "driving distance of approximately one hour or more" from an MTF. We asked providers how the remoteness of some patients affected treatment for this population, and we queried administrators about existing practices for ensuring access to high-quality care for remote service members. This chapter presents those perspectives.

Use of Telehealth with Remote Service Members

Most respondents ($n = 46$) reported that they provided or oversaw care for remote service members. However, less than one-quarter ($n = 10$) of these respondents had any experience using audio-only or video telehealth with remote service members prior to the pandemic. The majority of respondents ($n = 31$) told us that telehealth was not used with remote service members prior to the pandemic. One respondent described it as "simply forbidden," likely because telehealth visits were previously initiated between MTFs and not directly between patients and providers. Many reported that they aimed to schedule in-person visits with remote service members for when the service member planned to be at the installation. According to one provider/

administrator, "I think telehealth didn't even cross the minds of those guys [remote service members] as an option until COVID." One respondent told us that if remote patients were unable to drive to the MTF for their appointments, they might be referred to an intensive outpatient program or other higher level of care.

Although it was not the focus of our interviews, respondents who did use telehealth in some capacity with remote service members prior to the pandemic offered information about the model or circumstances under which they had delivered audio-only or video telehealth to this population. Respondents at an OCONUS MTF had used a direct-to-consumer model, in which service members in the field (for training or on deployment to a remote location) would receive virtual care from a provider located at the MTF. Meanwhile, some respondents at CONUS MTFs described a hub-and-spoke configuration for telehealth, in which the MTF provider would deliver care to a patient located at a regional, outlying, or other remote MTF. Although it was less common, several respondents at OCONUS and CONUS MTFs alike reported previous use of telehealth in ad hoc situations—for example, phone follow-up with a patient who had been referred to a private-sector provider but had not yet established a relationship with that new provider or video telehealth between MTFs to facilitate a patient evaluation. Such uses often served as temporary solutions to address barriers or to connect remote service members with a community provider or a new MTF for continuing care.

Use of Telehealth with Remote Service Members Following the Onset of the Pandemic

Although many MTF staff had already referred remote service members to private-sector providers (and thus delivered care to few remote patients), the onset of the pandemic did change the delivery of health care for many existing remote patients. All the respondents ($n = 10$) who described using telehealth with remote service members prior to the pandemic reported some continued use of telehealth with this population during the pandemic. Of the respondents who said they treated remote service members during the pandemic ($n = 46$), most ($n = 31$) told us that telehealth was helping to ameliorate access or transit barriers. They described telehealth as a critical means for remote service members to receive care when they might not have had other options. As one clinician recounted, "We have one individual that he had to drive two hours to get here and then two hours back home. There was nothing in his area where he lived. So being able to provide treatment virtually to him was like a lifesaver, you know?" Some even spoke of gravitating more readily to using telehealth with remote service members compared with non-remote service members.

Respondents who reported that telehealth alleviated access or transit barriers for remote service member patients at their MTF during the pandemic (n = 31) also reported varying degrees of telehealth use with this population. Several told us that they were using telehealth as "more of a stopgap" with remote service members, administering shorter sessions by phone or using the phone for safety checks between occasional in-person visits (n = 3). Several others said they were using telehealth to provide care for all their remote service member patients during the pandemic, generally describing full-length audio-only or video sessions with remote service members participating from home (n = 4). Others fell somewhere in between. Several respondents (n = 6) told us that telehealth increased continuity of care for remote service members, particularly while they were on missions, receiving dispositional follow-up, or transferring to another provider. One provider/administrator remarked, "[I've] seen them [remote service members] while on [temporary duty], mission, various locations, traveling. There was not a break then in service."

Still, among respondents who told us they treated remote service members (n = 46), nearly half (n = 19) said they were not using telehealth with all these patients. In some cases, respondents stated that telehealth with this population had been discouraged prior to the pandemic, and this continued to be the case for some or all remote service members. Respondents also mentioned related barriers, such as concerns about safety and the need for National Guard or reserve service members to be on active duty to receive treatment at an MTF. At least one respondent explained that limited staffing for telehealth at their MTF reduced telehealth possibilities for remote service members.

Potential of Telehealth to Increase Access to and Continuity of Care for Remote Service Members

More than half of respondents across all the MTFs in our sample acknowledged the unique value of greater use of telehealth with remote service members ($n = 36$). Providers who had experience treating this population prior to the pandemic suggested that requiring in-person visits for remote service members was costly to the military, time-consuming and disruptive to the service member's life and duties, and detrimental to the quality of care delivery because it fragmented the course of therapy and resulted in poorer access to care. One respondent made the following plea:

> I want to really advocate that the Army or military consider not having services be location-based, which they are. So, right now, all the infrastructure is based on where is the clinic, how appointments get made, and there is a lot of cumbersome infrastructure and logistics right now.
>
> But to look at, can a service member come into the military, their first behavioral health visit is in person and if they connect well, they get an episode of care, things are good. Then they [experience a permanent change of station], go [on temporary duty], get deployed, need another episode of care. Can they connect back to that same provider virtually and have continuity over the course of their career potentially or at least to a greater extent? . . . Because [when] . . . you know the patient history, you know what the good/bad looks like for them, you can treat them much quicker. And you already have the established trust. So, I think there is a lot of good that can come from doing business that way.

Nearly half of the respondents who provided treatment to remote service members reported that distance was an obstacle for these patients and that telehealth had the potential to help ($n = 20$). Nearly one-quarter of respondents who provided treatment to remote service members commented that they felt telehealth had the potential to improve continuity of care for remote service members—particularly those on missions or experiencing a permanent change of station—or to facilitate administrative oversight for remote service members referred to community network providers ($n = 10$). Several also said they felt that telehealth could save the MHS time and money (e.g., on medical evacuations, travel expenses, cost of care, work interruptions; $n = 6$).

Barriers to Using Telehealth with Remote Service Members

Providers also described barriers that the MHS would need to address if the potential benefits of telehealth are to be realized for remote service members.

MTF Staffing and Referral Policies

Perhaps the greatest barrier to increased use of telehealth with remote service members was that most providers referred these patients to the community for BH care. MTFs are typically staffed to support non-remote service members only, and it is standard practice to refer most remote service members to private-sector providers in their communities. Most respondents across all the MTFs in our sample told us that telehealth was simply not used for all remote service members prior to the pandemic ($n = 31$). In some cases, it was specifically disallowed. According to one respondent,

> For [the Army Substance Use Disorder Clinical Care program], since a large proportion of our folks are command-directed (so if I get a call from reservists, and they live in a rural area), our regulations say they have to be [provided with a permanent change of station] closer to an MTF so that they can participate in an evidence-based treatment.

Particularly at the MTFs where telehealth for remote service members was not permitted prior to the pandemic, some respondents told us that this population was to be treated in person even during the pandemic, while others said they were uncertain about the policy on the use of telehealth with remote service members. One provider/administrator said, "There wasn't any telehealth option [for remote service members]. As of now, that hasn't changed. I don't know if it will be changing or not." In general, there was a sense among several of our respondents that MTFs were not staffed to adequately serve all remote service members and, thus, it was unclear how to determine which remote service members (if any) might be eligible for telehealth services.

Treating High-Risk or High-Severity Patients

Some of the challenges that staff faced in using telehealth with local patients were the same or more pronounced with remote service members. Concerns about patient risk (e.g., suicidal ideation) among remote service members or being "nervous about treating somebody in the middle of nowhere" were mentioned by several respondents ($n = 5$) across half of MTFs. These individuals pointed to a lack of clear protocol for handling patient emergencies for individuals located far from the MTF, suggesting that there was "no clear chain of command." Providers also expressed concern about treating patients across service branches, suggesting that communication is fragmented, and it is difficult to know how to complete a patient profile or follow other procedures for patients in other service branches.

Summary

This chapter examined the use of telehealth with remote service members and the perspectives of BH staff on the benefits of these modalities and barriers to their use at the MTFs in our sample. The majority of respondents reported that telehealth was not used with remote service members prior to the pandemic, but those who had used it with this population reported that they continued to do so in some capacity during the pandemic.

Across all MTFs, more than half of respondents acknowledged the value of using telehealth with remote service members, including its potential to increase access and continuity of care. Barriers to the wider use of telehealth with remote service members included a tendency for these patients be seen by private-sector providers, lack of MTF staff to deliver telehealth to these service members, and concerns about telehealth use with patients at high risk or with more-severe symptoms.

CHAPTER EIGHT

Summary and Recommendations

This report described military BH staff perspectives on telehealth following the onset of the COVID-19 pandemic. We conducted analyses of semi-structured interviews with 52 BH providers and administrators from ten MTFs approximately six months into the pandemic. Interviews covered a range of topics related to providing BH care to service members with a focus on the use of telehealth to treat PTSD, depression, and SUDs during the pandemic and the factors associated with this use. We conducted qualitative data analyses to identify key themes from our interviews. This chapter explains the strengths and limitations of our approach, summarizes key findings drawn from military BH staff perceptions of telehealth, and presents policy recommendations based on these findings.

Strengths and Limitations

We note some limitations in our methodological approach. First, we interviewed a small number of staff across ten MTFs, and our findings represent their perceptions on the use of telehealth in BH care delivery. Although we selected MTFs in a way that maximized variability in BH staff perspectives, the ten MTFs in our study might not reflect the diversity of telehealth practices and perspectives across the MHS. Furthermore, we identified staff to interview in collaboration with key contacts at each MTF. Key contacts were asked to identify several potential participants using the guidance we provided (e.g., eligible to participate, individuals drawn from across clinics and provider types). This may have resulted in some bias if key contacts were more likely to identify individuals perceived as higher-performing in some way (e.g., telehealth competence, delivery of evidence-based BH care).

Second, there were some limitations associated with our data collection approach. To ensure that staff felt comfortable speaking frankly, we did not record our interviews. Instead, we took transcription-style notes, and we may have missed some exact quotations. We developed the interview guide prior to the onset of the pandemic, and it was not exclusively focused on telehealth. Thus, this report might not offer a full account of staff experiences and perspectives on telehealth (e.g., whether providers were delivering telehealth from home). Third, our interviews were conducted between July and October 2020 (but predominantly in August and September); this timing could be associated with some variability in perspectives, depending on the state of the pandemic at particular MTFs at the time of our interviews. Furthermore, our rapid coding process, which involved assigning a large number of thematic codes, meant that we did not formally "double-code" interviews or compute a formal intercoder reliability statistic (although we did use a team of three members to audit and cross-check the coding).[1] Finally, we present findings based on the perceptions and experiences of BH staff at the time of our interviews. We did not conduct a formal evaluation to document existing MHS policies on telehealth, the adequacy of MHS telehealth infrastructure and capabilities, or the availability and adequacy of telehealth training and clinical tools.

Despite these limitations, our approach had several strengths. First, we conducted interviews rapidly after the onset of the pandemic. This provided a unique opportunity to capture staff experiences when the need for and use of telehealth options were especially heightened. Moreover, qualitative data collection allowed us to capture more-nuanced responses that might not have been captured through quantitative data collection. Finally, our sample included providers and administrators from across service branches, clinic types, and provider types drawn from ten diverse MTFs, increasing the variety of experiences captured in the data. Staff represented a rich diversity of telehealth experience, from seasoned administrators who had been working to implement and refine telehealth practices for many years to telehealth-naïve providers who may not have otherwise ever used telehealth

---

[1] This is common in qualitative rapid analyses, including recent studies of emerging changes in clinical practice during the COVID-19 pandemic. See Uscher-Pines et al., 2020.

if the extreme circumstances of the pandemic not called for this modality to ensure continuity of care. Thus, the perspectives described in this report offer uniquely valuable information that the MHS can leverage as it readies for a more intentional and organized effort toward firmly establishing telehealth at an enterprise scale.

The remainder of this chapter highlights the main findings from the report, followed by recommendations for how the MHS can continue to integrate telehealth to meet the BH needs of service members.

Key Findings

Use of Telehealth Increased Dramatically Following the Onset of the Pandemic, but It Varied Within and Across MTFs, and Many MTFs Were Already Returning to In-Person Care

Nearly all respondents noted a dramatic shift from in-person care to audio-only or video telehealth or to a combination of in-person and telehealth modalities early in the pandemic. Transitions at the pandemic's onset ranged from a complete cessation of services at one MTF to a rapid transition by all providers to offering audio-only or video telehealth services for most patients at another MTF. Nearly all respondents reported using audio-only telehealth, but less than half reported using video telehealth. Staff varied in how they used audio-only telehealth. Some providers described using it for shorter visits or check-ins, while others mentioned attempting to deliver full-length sessions. More than half of providers reported at least some integration of mobile apps into their BH care delivery. There was also variation in the proportion of telehealth relative to in-person care during the pandemic. Several providers said they delivered mostly in-person care, while others teleworked part- or full-time and made audio-only or video telehealth calls from personal devices, laptops, work computers, or designated video telehealth equipment.

There was variation in intentions to continue offering telehealth, ranging from a return to in-person care delivery to efforts to sustain or expand telehealth use, as well as combinations of these approaches. At the time of our interviews, half of respondents across all MTFs told us they were getting "back to normal." However, respondents at six MTFs told us that in-person treatment was "no longer the default," suggesting that telehealth could play an ongoing role in BH care provision after the pandemic.

Most Providers Were Open to Using Video Telehealth, but Widespread Technological Challenges and a Lack of Clear Policy Guidance Impeded More-Frequent Use

Most providers were not using video telehealth at the time of our interviews. However, more than three-quarters of these providers expressed an interest in using it in the future. Among the providers who did report video telehealth use, just over half expressed an openness to continued use of this modality. Nearly all providers were using audio-only telehealth at the time of our interviews, yet only about a quarter indicated that they were open to continuing to use it. One-third mentioned that they were open to either continued or future use of mobile apps. Reasons for low uptake of video telehealth were most commonly related to technology. Nearly all respondents expressed concerns about having adequate technology to support telehealth, such as computing equipment, bandwidth, technical support, video telehealth platforms, and data security. Such issues were particularly problematic for those attempting to use video telehealth, although equipment was also a barrier for some using audio-only telehealth. Respondents characterized existing video telehealth platforms as unreliable. Some staff also expressed concern about the security of various platforms and models of care delivery for video telehealth. Finally, nearly all staff described administrative and logistical barriers to implementing telehealth, such as problems scheduling appointments while teleworking, documenting sessions, exchanging paperwork, and monitoring patients' symptoms. Staff from most MTFs expressed frustration with bureaucratic barriers, unclear guidance, or a perceived lack of support for audio-only and video telehealth at the MTF or DHA level.

Staff Expressed Concerns About Using Telehealth with High-Risk Patients, Those Diagnosed with PTSD or SUD, and Those Receiving Group Therapy

Nearly all respondents shared opinions about the appropriateness of telehealth for specific patient populations or types of visits (e.g., group versus individual therapy). Most reported that high-risk patients were typically seen in person during the pandemic.

About half of respondents expressed concerns about using telehealth to treat high-risk patients or patients with high symptom severity. These concerns were more pronounced when it came to audio-only telehealth as opposed to video telehealth, with an inability to assess certain symptoms among the reasons. Nearly one-third of staff expressed at least some concern regarding telehealth for PTSD, and nearly one-fifth expressed at least some concern regarding telehealth for SUD. These staff indicated that an inability to assess patients for clinical deterioration during treatment sessions for PTSD or for, patients with SUD, signs or symptoms associated with recent use or withdrawal from substances played a large role in their concerns. We did not hear serious concerns about using telehealth with non–high-risk patients with depression.

Providers often cited the unreliability of telehealth technology as a contributing barrier. About one-quarter of respondents mentioned that group therapy sessions had stopped since the onset of the pandemic, and about one-fifth expressed concerns about using audio-only or video telehealth to deliver effective group therapy. Relatedly, about one-third of respondents across nearly all MTFs shared concerns about using telehealth to conduct intake assessments or suggested that it should be used with established patients only.

Staff Indicated That Both Patients and Providers Needed More Orientation to Telehealth

Just over half of staff reported that they believed patients liked telehealth, largely citing the increased convenience. For example, patients were able to save on driving time, get care even if they lacked access to transportation, and obtain medication refills over the phone rather than needing to miss work to attend in-person appointments. However, nearly one-third of respondents said that some patients disliked telehealth and preferred to receive in-person care. Reasons included a lack of trust in the security of audio-only or video telehealth technology and difficulty using the technology. A third of staff described a "learning curve" as they gradually became more comfortable with telehealth modalities. Facing technological barriers in the absence of technical support, training, or clear guidance, providers stated that it took time "to get familiar with the equipment" and requirements for telehealth. Similarly, more than one-third of respondents from most MTFs referenced a patient learning curve, noting that patients needed orientation to ensure that telehealth visits were as effective as in-person visits. Providers also described a need to socialize their patients to telehealth etiquette and protocols, as well as to establish procedures for sharing information about technological requirements with patients by email or text message.

Staff Believed That Telehealth Was a Promising Approach for Service Members Who Lived Far from an MTF but Reported Barriers to Using Telehealth with These Patients

The majority of respondents reported that they did not use telehealth with remote service members prior to the pandemic. However, more than half from across all MTFs acknowledged the unique value of using telehealth with these service members, including increased access and continuity of care. Respondents particularly recognized the benefits for service members who were located one hour or more from an MTF, on temporary duty orders, in geographically separated units, on deployment to remote OCONUS locations, and in transition because of a permanent change of station. They suggested that, in these cases, remote service members might have otherwise encountered too many challenges to seek treatment at an MTF and would likely have experienced a temporary disruption in care.

Many staff typically referred remote service members to private-sector providers prior to the pandemic and thus delivered care to few remote patients. Those who did serve this population reported that telehealth typically was not used, and many described continuing barriers to its use *during* the pandemic. Although most of these respondents said that telehealth had ameliorated barriers for one or more remote service member patients, this seemed to be more of an exception than a rule. Nearly half said that telehealth was not always used with all remote service members during the pandemic. However, there was broad recognition that existing MTF staffing and referral practices did not support ongoing use of telehealth with this population. Concerns about treating high-risk or high-symptom-severity patients were also mentioned as a possible barrier.

Recommendations

In this section, we provide recommendations for how the MHS can continue to expand efforts to integrate and sustain use of telehealth in delivery of BH care. These recommendations were developed based on the findings from our staff interviews.

Recommendation 1. Develop Policy Guidance on the Use of Telehealth for Patients with Behavioral Health Conditions

Staff expressed a desire for clear policy guidance on telehealth practice. DHA typically codifies policy guidance in the form of procedural instructions or procedural manuals but, as of March 2021, it had not developed such guidance for telehealth. A national survey of licensed psychologists found that providers in settings with supportive organizational policies were more likely to use telehealth during the pandemic (Pierce et al., 2021). Policy guidance should address the technology requirements for successful telehealth delivery and provide guidance on expectations for high-quality treatment. For example, DHA might specify cases in which audio-only telehealth is allowable. Staff and providers should also be instructed on minimum information collection requirements for telehealth patients. There is a need to standardize policy guidance and clinical guidelines on the safe treatment of patients across the MHS. Allowances might be made for MTF- or command-level variation in telehealth implementation, provided that there is adherence to minimum legal and regulatory requirements. Because the security of telehealth systems is a concern among both providers and patients, MHS guidance regarding best practices for data security and privacy would be particularly valuable in increasing comfort with telehealth and facilitating its adoption. DHA released interim guidance in March and August 2020 (Place, 2020; Cordts, 2020), along with standards of practice for behavioral health during the pandemic period (DHA, 2020). The rapid release of these documents highlights the evolving nature of the pandemic response.

Recommendation 2. Develop and Implement a Strategic Plan to Ensure That Providers Have Adequate Technology to Support Video Telehealth

Across all the MTFs in our study, staff reported technological infrastructure barriers to telehealth adoption. In some cases, the absence of adequate technology meant that providers could not even attempt to deliver video telehealth. In others, poor connectivity, inadequate bandwidth, and difficulty using telehealth platforms posed challenges, slowing the adoption of telehealth. It should be noted that our findings reflect the perceptions of BH staff; we did not conduct a formal evaluation to document the adequacy of existing telehealth infrastructure and capabilities in the MHS. However, our findings suggest that the MHS should develop and implement a strategic plan to ensure that providers have adequate technology to deliver video telehealth.

According to the Office of the National Coordinator for Health Information Technology, the technical infrastructure requirements for telehealth include reliable access to broadband internet with enough bandwidth to support video data transmission, as well as access to technical support staff to assist with implementation and ongoing technical troubleshooting, as needed (Office of the National Coordinator for Health Information Technology, 2019). Staff need appropriate office space and necessary equipment, such as computers with cameras and user-friendly telehealth platforms (Pineau et al., 2006; Tsiouris et al., 2020).

To ensure adequate broadband access, the MHS could evaluate existing internet access at MTFs and develop minimum access and bandwidth standards. At the MTF level, command leadership might elect to purchase increased broadband or arrange for secure wireless internet to facilitate the flexible use of physical space. It might also be beneficial to develop a specialized method for providers to connect with patients who live in military congregate housing. Improved internet access in military barracks could increase the reliability of video telehealth. It might also be useful to designate a physical space for telehealth appointments in the event that service members are unable to find a private location for an audio or video call.

Ideally, the MHS would adopt a user-friendly, reliable, and secure telehealth platform that is compatible with multiple types of devices and adaptable to both individual and group treatment. It might be beneficial to first evaluate existing platforms to identify potential improvements to meet these needs. For example, the Veterans Health Administration developed VA Video Connect, an encrypted HIPAA-compliant platform for video telehealth (Rosen et al., 2021). There might be platforms in use within the MHS that could be adopted for telehealth services, or the MHS might choose a novel platform. In any case, the selected platform should be optimized for both individual and group treatment. If possible, it should be accessible to patients and providers from mobile devices or computers. Staff should be able to access the system both while on site at the MTF and while teleworking. Considerations should be made for how to support document signing, symptom monitoring, and the exchange of paperwork (e.g., therapy materials) either within the telehealth platform or separately.

Recommendation 3. Provide Clinical and Technical Training on the Use of Telehealth

Recommendation 3a. Provide Training on the Clinical Aspects of Telehealth

Although most staff did not specifically request additional training, they expressed concerns about using audio-only or video telehealth in a variety of clinical situations. Although we did not conduct a formal review of the adequacy of training for MHS providers on the clinical aspects of telehealth, staff discomfort suggests the need for additional training. Earlier, we recommended the development of formal policy guidance on telehealth (in the form of a procedural instruction or procedural manual), along with clinical protocols. Here, we recommend that providers receive additional training on the clinical aspects of telehealth that would allow them to implement formal policy guidance, clinical protocols, and treatment decisions.

For example, a lack of identified competencies might have left providers feeling underprepared for differences in risk management in a telehealth environment and thus reluctant to use telehealth with at-risk patients. These types of clinical situations can be managed well using telehealth with adequate provider training and measurable, evidence-based frameworks for telehealth competencies (Hilty et al., 2015; Johnson, 2014; Maheu et al., 2017, 2018). For example, in 2017, the Coalition for Technology in Behavioral Sciences developed interprofessional telebehavioral health competencies to improve the quality and safety of care through the use of standardized training (Maheu et al., 2018). These competencies are organized into seven general domains and three levels of expertise for different segments of the BH workforce (i.e., novice clinician, proficient clinician, or authority/expert). The seven domains are as follows: (1) clinical evaluation and care, with the subdomains of cultural competence and diversity, documentation, and administrative procedures; (2) the virtual environment and telepresence; (3) technology; (4) legal and regulatory issues; (5) evidence-based and ethical practice, with the subdomain social media; (6) mobile health and apps; and (7) telepractice development (Maheu et al., 2018). The domains are further categorized into 51 telehealth objectives according to the three competency levels.

Training that targets the specific concerns and competency levels of providers would increase comfort, knowledge, and skills and would potentially improve attitudes toward telehealth. Providers might also need support in identifying clinical scenarios that are appropriate for telehealth. Standardized, empirically based criteria for making this determination could also support clinical decisionmaking. Structured guidance could help providers assess patients based on their diagnoses, level of symptom severity, type and degree of risk (e.g., suicidal ideation, recent hospitalization), stage of treatment, and type of treatment being delivered to determine the appropriate integration of telehealth. In addition, providers would benefit from materials to socialize patients to both the technical and clinical aspects of telehealth.

Finally, providers will need training in the mechanics of delivering evidence-based treatment using video telehealth, particularly psychotherapy. A survey of telebehavioral health experts indicated a need for guidance in adapting evidence-based practices to a telehealth setting, and there have been several telehealth case studies of solutions for delivering evidence-based BH care to active-duty service members at MTFs (Waltman et al., 2020). Successful adaptations included using screen-sharing technology, incorporating other technology-based resources (such as mobile applications), and using web-based methods to securely administer outcome tracking measures. Training on these and other adaptations could facilitate stronger interest and confidence in using telehealth modalities to deliver evidence-based care.

Recommendation 3b. Provide Technical Training and Support for Telehealth

Staff expressed a desire for access to technical support and training in telehealth implementation. This was consistent with findings from studies of civilian providers, who reported technical difficulties as their most common concern despite overall positive attitudes toward telehealth (Connolly et al., 2020). Comprehensive training in telehealth competencies could obviate some of these concerns, but targeted technical training in video telehealth could further increase familiarity and comfort. For example, to address providers' concerns about missing important nonverbal behavioral cues, training could show them how to direct patients to adjust their camera and lighting to provide a better view (Connolly et al., 2020). We did not conduct a review of existing training available to MHS providers on the technical aspects of telehealth delivery. We note that two brief (45-minute) trainings are available to MHS providers on the basics of telehealth, with one geared toward providers and another toward "presenters" (i.e., support personnel who facilitate connections between providers and patients) (DHA, undated b, undated a). Our interviews did not document the use of these particular training resources or whether providers viewed available training as adequate if they had taken it. Yet it was clear that providers saw a need for additional assistance with the technological aspects of telehealth.

Finally, it might be worthwhile to identify existing IT support staff and conduct an initial assessment of the potential scalability of their capabilities at a given MTF. And at the system level, there might be a need to increase IT staffing to ensure that there is someone on site at each MTF to troubleshoot or provide in-home assistance (for providers who are teleworking).

Summary

Preliminary evidence indicates that the COVID-19 pandemic increased demand for BH care among service members and their dependents who are eligible for TRICARE, just as it did for civilian populations. At the same time, the adaptations required to continue delivering care might have affected MHS efforts to improve service members' access to BH care and the quality of care they received. Telehealth filled a gap for some MTFs and providers early on in the pandemic, but there was some uncertainty about its future utility at the time of our interviews. The findings and recommendations in this report illustrate how telehealth can—with the appropriate training, technology, guidance, and policies—increase access to BH care and help the MHS better meet the needs of all service members.

Interview Guide

Structured Questions

Interviewer: Confirm the following information about the participant before the interview begins. Ask the participant these questions only if the information cannot be confirmed otherwise (e.g., can confirm military branch by the base location of the interview).

Military service branch:

- a. Army
- b. Navy
- c. Marines
- d. Air Force

Status:

- a. Active component
- b. National Guard, full time
- c. National Guard, part time
- d. Reserve
- e. DoD government civilian
- f. Contractor (Note: Contractors are ineligible for the study. Please thank them for their time and do not interview.)

Rank (if applicable):

- a. C-1, E-1–E-4
- b. E-5–E-9
- c. O-1–O-3
- d. O-4–O-8

Do you have clinical role, administrative role, or both?

    a.   Clinical

    b.   Administrative

    c.   Both

Do you currently treat service members with. . . ? *(Circle all that apply.)*

    a.   PTSD

    b.   Depression

    c.   SUD

Which types of clinics do you work in? *(Circle all that apply.)*

    a.   Primary care

    b.   Mental health specialty care

    c.   SUD specialty care

    d.   Integrated mental health/SUD care program

    e.   Other: _____

What type of provider? *(Interviewer: Circle the one that aligns most closely.)*

    a.   Psychiatrist

    b.   Psychologist

    c.   M.S.W./M.A. counselor

    d.   SUD counselor

    e.   Primary care practitioner

    f.   Other: _____

Use of Evidence-Based Practices

Interviewer: Focus on current practice but understand pre-pandemic experiences/perceptions.

    a.   *[For providers who have delivered care for PTSD]* What treatment approaches have you used to treat patients with PTSD? Please describe your primary treatment approach.

        i.   Therapy approaches (e.g., trauma-focused cognitive behavioral therapy, such as eye movement desensitization and reprocessing, cognitive processing therapy, prolonged exposure, or stress inoculation training)

    ii.   Medications prescribed (e.g., SSRIs/SNRIs)

    iii. Assess delivery of evidence-based practices (e.g., homework assigned, number of sessions, structure of treatment, assess symptoms during treatment)

b.   *[For providers who have delivered care for depression]* What treatment approaches have you used to treat patients with depression? Please describe your primary treatment approach.

    i.   Therapy approaches (e.g., cognitive behavioral therapy, interpersonal therapy, problem-solving therapy)

    ii.   Medications prescribed (e.g., SSRIs/SNRIs)

    iii. Assess delivery of evidence-based practices (e.g., homework assigned, number of sessions, structure of treatment, assess symptoms during treatment)

c.   *[For providers who have delivered care for SUD]* What treatment approaches have you used to treat patients with SUD? Please describe your primary treatment approach.

    i.   Therapy approaches (e.g., cognitive behavioral therapy)

    ii.   Medications prescribed (e.g., Naloxone)

    iii. Assess delivery of evidence-based practices (e.g., homework assigned, number of sessions, structure of treatment, assess symptoms during treatment)

d.   *[For administrators]* How do you assess the types of treatments that providers are using to treat PTSD, depression, and SUD and the degree to which the treatments are evidence-based?

    i. *Prompts:* provider training, chart review, live or taped observation

Barriers and Facilitators to Delivering Evidence-Based Treatments for PTSD, Depression, and SUD

a. *[For providers]* What have you found helps or supports you in being able to deliver evidence-based treatment for PTSD, depression, and SUD?

b. *[For providers]* What gets in the way of your ability to deliver evidence-based treatment for PTSD, depression, and SUD?

    i. *Prompts (structural barriers):* High caseloads, availability of appointments, lack of leadership support for evidence-based practices, handling institutional demands for disciplinary action versus therapeutic response (for SUD)?

    ii. *Prompts (provider barriers):* Lack of training, prefer other treatments over evidence-based practices

    iii. *Prompts (patient/service member barriers):* Service member duties, stigma

    iv. Note any unique issues for SUD or difference between treatment for mental health conditions versus SUD

c. *[For providers]* What recommendations do you have to overcome these barriers?

d. *[For administrators]* What have you found helps or supports the providers you oversee in being able to deliver evidence-based treatment for PTSD, depression, and SUD?

Perceptions of Telebehavioral Health Options

a. *[For providers]* What experience do you have with using telehealth to treat behavioral health conditions like PTSD, depression, and SUD? Telehealth options include providing treatment via videoconference or telephone or working with patients to use mobile apps to treat or manage symptoms.

    i. *If no experience, assess reasons* (e.g., structural resources not present, viewed as not helpful or feasible).

ii. *If experience, assess perceptions* (i.e., positive, negative, barriers to use, apps and websites used).

b. *[For administrators]* In your administrative role, how do you view telehealth options to treat behavioral health conditions like PTSD, depression, and SUD? Telehealth options include providing treatment via videoconference or telephone or working with patients to use mobile apps to treat or manage symptoms.

Considerations for Service Members Who Reside in Areas Remote from Care

a. *[For providers]* Do you see service members who reside far from the MTF? How does this affect your treatment for these service members?

b. *[For providers]* If a service member resides far from the MTF, does this affect whether you use telehealth options in their treatment?

c. *[For administrators]* What administrative practices are in place to help ensure access to high-quality care to service members who reside far from the MTF?

Closing
Do you have any other comments on the topics we discussed today?

Abbreviations

BH	behavioral health
BHDP	Behavioral Health Data Portal
CONUS	continental United States
COVID-19	coronavirus disease 2019
DHA	Defense Health Agency
DoD	U.S. Department of Defense
HIPAA	Health Insurance Portability and Accountability Act
IT	information technology
MHS	Military Health System
M.S.W.	master's in social work
MTF	military treatment facility
OCONUS	outside the continental United States
PTSD	posttraumatic stress disorder
SNRI	serotonin-norepinephrine reuptake inhibitor
SSRI	selective serotonin reuptake inhibitor
SUD	substance use disorder
VA	U.S. Department of Veterans Affairs

References

Acierno, Ron, Rebecca Knapp, Peter Tuerk, Amanda K. Gilmore, Carl Lejuez, Kenneth Ruggiero, Wendy Muzzy, Leonard Egede, Melba A. Hernandez-Tejada, and Edna B. Foa, "A Non-Inferiority Trial of Prolonged Exposure for Posttraumatic Stress Disorder: In Person Versus Home-Based Telehealth," *Behaviour Research and Therapy,* Vol. 89, February 2017, pp. 57–65.

Bashshur, Rashid L., Gary W. Shannon, Noura Bashshur, and Peter M. Yellowlees, "The Empirical Evidence for Telemedicine Interventions in Mental Disorders," *Telemedicine Journal and E-Health,* Vol. 22, No. 2, February 2016, pp. 87–113.

Benavides-Vaello, Sandra, Anne Strode, and Beth C. Sheeran, "Using Technology in the Delivery of Mental Health and Substance Abuse Treatment in Rural Communities: A Review," *Journal of Behavioral Health Services and Research,* Vol. 40, No. 1, January 2013, pp. 111–120.

Berryhill, Micha Blake, Nathan Culmer, Nelle Williams, Anne Halli-Tierney, Alex Betancourt, Hannah Roberts, and Michael King, "Videoconferencing Psychotherapy and Depression: A Systematic Review," *Telemedicine Journal and E-Health,* Vol. 25, No. 6, June 2019, pp. 435–446.

Bolton, A. J., and D. S. Dorstyn, "Telepsychology for Posttraumatic Stress Disorder: A Systematic Review," *Journal of Telemedicine and Telecare,* Vol. 21, No. 5, July 2015, pp. 254–267.

Breslau, Joshua, Melissa L. Finucane, Alicia R. Locker, Matthew D. Baird, Elizabeth A. Roth, and Rebecca L. Collins, "A Longitudinal Study of Psychological Distress in the United States Before and During the COVID-19 Pandemic," *Preventive Medicine,* Vol. 143, February 2021, article 106362.

Brown, Ryan Andrew, Grant N. Marshall, Joshua Breslau, Coreen Farris, Karen Chan Osilla, Harold Alan Pincus, Teague Ruder, Phoenix Voorhies, Dionne Barnes-Proby, Katherine Pfrommer, et al., *Access to Behavioral Health Care for Geographically Remote Service Members and Dependents in the U.S.,* Santa Monica, Calif.: RAND Corporation, RR-578-OSD, 2015. As of September 7, 2021:
https://www.rand.org/pubs/research_reports/RR578.html

Centers for Medicare and Medicaid Services, "Trump Administration Makes Sweeping Regulatory Changes to Help U.S. Healthcare System Address COVID-19 Patient Surge," press release, March 30, 2020. As of September 7, 2021:
https://www.cms.gov/newsroom/press-releases/trump-administration-makes-sweeping-regulatory-changes-help-us-healthcare-system-address-covid-19

Chen, Justin A., Wei-Jean Chung, Sarah K. Young, Margaret C. Tuttle, Michelle B. Collins, Sarah L. Darghouth, Regina Longley, Raymond Levy, Mahdi Razafsha, Jeffrey C. Kerner, et al., "COVID-19 and Telepsychiatry: Early Outpatient Experiences and Implications for the Future," *General Hospital Psychiatry*, Vol. 66, September–October 2020, pp. 89–95.

Cohen, Gregory H., David S. Fink, Laura Sampson, and Sandro Galea, "Mental Health Among Reserve Component Military Service Members and Veterans," *Epidemiologic Reviews*, Vol. 37, No. 1, 2015, pp. 7–22.

Connolly, Samantha L., Christopher J. Miller, Jan A. Lindsay, and Mark S. Bauer, "A Systematic Review of Providers' Attitudes Toward Telemental Health via Videoconferencing," *Clinical Psychology: Science and Practice*, Vol. 27, No. 2, June 2020, article e12311.

Cordts, Paul R., Defense Health Agency, "Interim Virtual Health (VH) Guidance During COVID-19 Pandemic Response," memorandum to market directors, Falls Church, Va., August 8, 2020.

Coughtrey, Anna E., and Nancy Pistrang, "The Effectiveness of Telephone-Delivered Psychological Therapies for Depression and Anxiety: A Systematic Review," *Journal of Telemedicine and Telecare*, Vol. 24, No. 2, February 2018, pp. 65–74.

Czeisler, Mark É., Rashon I. Lane, Emiko Petrosky, Joshua F. Wiley, Aleta Christensen, Rashid Njai, Matthew D. Weaver, Rebecca Robbins, Elise R. Facer-Childs, Laura K. Barger, et al., "Mental Health, Substance Use, and Suicidal Ideation During the COVID-19 Pandemic—United States, June 24–30, 2020," *Morbidity and Mortality Weekly Report*, Vol. 69, No. 32, August 14, 2020, pp. 1049–1057.

Defense Health Agency, "DHA—US444-DHA Virtual Health Provider Training," Falls Church, Va., undated a.

———, "DHA—US445-DHA Virtual Health Presenter Training," undated b.

———, "mHealth Clinical Integration," webpage, undated c. As of September 7, 2021:
https://health.mil/About-MHS/OASDHA/Defense-Health-Agency/Operations/Clinical-Support-Division/Connected-Health/mHealth-Clinical-Integration

———, *Military Health System, Virtual Behavioral Health Guidelines*, version 1.0, Falls Church, Va., April 4, 2020.

Defense Health Agency Procedural Instruction 6490.02, *Behavioral Health (BH) Treatment and Outcomes Monitoring*, July 12, 2018.

DHA—*See* Defense Health Agency.

Docherty, Mary, Brigitta Spaeth-Rublee, Deborah Scharf, Erin K. Ferenchick, Jennifer Humensky, Matthew L. Goldman, Henry Chung, and Harold Alan Pincus, "How Practices Can Advance the Implementation of Integrated Care in the COVID-19 Era," Commonwealth Fund, November 17, 2020. As of September 7, 2021:
https://www.commonwealthfund.org/publications/issue-briefs/2020/nov/practices-advance-implementation-integrated-care-covid

DoD—*See* U.S. Department of Defense.

Duncan, Greg J., "When to Promote, and When to Avoid, a Population Perspective," *Demography*, Vol. 45, No. 4, November 2008, pp. 763–784.

Ettman, Catherine K., Salma M. Abdalla, Gregory H. Cohen, Laura Sampson, Patrick M. Vivier, and Sandro Galea, "Prevalence of Depression Symptoms in US Adults Before and During the COVID-19 Pandemic," *JAMA Network Open*, Vol. 3, No. 9, September 2, 2020, article e2019686.

Evans, Arthur C., Jr., CEO, American Psychological Association, letter to Secretary of Defense Mark T. Esper, October 16, 2020. As of September 7, 2021:
https://www.apa.org/news/press/releases/2020/10/letter-mental-health-access-tricare.pdf

Ferguson, Jacqueline M., Josephine Jacobs, Maria Yefimova, Liberty Greene, Leonie Heyworth, and Donna M. Zulman, "Virtual Care Expansion in the Veterans Health Administration During the COVID-19 Pandemic: Clinical Services and Patient Characteristics Associated with Utilization," *Journal of the American Medical Informatics Association*, Vol. 28, No. 3, March 2021, pp. 453–462.

Greenbaum, Zara, "How Well Is Telepsychology Working?" *Monitor on Psychology*, Vol. 51, No. 5, July 2020. As of September 7, 2021:
https://www.apa.org/monitor/2020/07/cover-telepsychology

Gros, Daniel F., Leslie A. Morland, Carolyn J. Greene, Ron Acierno, Martha Strachan, Leonard E. Egede, Peter W. Tuerk, Hugh Myrick, and B. Christopher Frueh, "Delivery of Evidence-Based Psychotherapy via Video Telehealth," *Journal of Psychopathology and Behavioral Assessment*, Vol. 35, No. 4, 2013, pp. 506–521.

Health Resources and Services Administration, "Behavioral Health Workforce Projections," webpage, December 2020. As of September 7, 2021:
https://bhw.hrsa.gov/data-research/projecting-health-workforce-supply-demand/behavioral-health

Hepner, Kimberly A., Ryan Andrew Brown, Carol P. Roth, Teague Ruder, and Harold Alan Pincus, *Behavioral Health Care in the Military Health System: Access and Quality for Remote Service Members*, Santa Monica, Calif.: RAND Corporation, RR-2788-OSD, 2021. As of September 7, 2021:
https://www.rand.org/pubs/research_reports/RR2788.html

Hepner, Kimberly A., Carol P. Roth, Elizabeth M. Sloss, Susan M. Paddock, Praise O. Iyiewuare, Martha J. Timmer, and Harold Alan Pincus, *Quality of Care for PTSD and Depression in the Military Health System: Final Report*, Santa Monica, Calif.: RAND Corporation, RR-1542-OSD, 2017. As of September 7, 2021:
https://www.rand.org/pubs/research_reports/RR1542.html

Hilty, Donald M., Allison Crawford, John Teshima, Steven Chan, Nadiya Sunderji, Peter M. Yellowlees, Greg Kramer, Patrick O'Neill, Chris Fore, John Luo, and Su-Ting Li, "A Framework for Telepsychiatric Training and E-Health: Competency-Based Education, Evaluation and Implications," *International Review of Psychiatry*, Vol. 27, No. 6, 2015, pp. 569–592.

Hummer, Justin, Kimberly A. Hepner, Carol P. Roth, Ryan Andrew Brown, Jessica L. Sousa, Teague Ruder, and Harold Alan Pincus, *Behavioral Health Care for National Guard and Reserve Service Members from the Military Health System*, Santa Monica, Calif.: RAND Corporation, RR-A421-1, 2021. As of September 22, 2021:
https://www.rand.org/pubs/research_reports/RRA421-1.html

Johnson, Gerald R., "Toward Uniform Competency Standards in Telepsychology: A Proposed Framework for Canadian Psychologists," *Canadian Psychology*, Vol. 55, No. 4, November 2014, pp. 291–302.

King, Van L., Kenneth B. Stoller, Michael Kidorf, Kori Kindbom, Steven Hursh, Thomas Brady, and Robert K. Brooner, "Assessing the Effectiveness of an Internet-Based Videoconferencing Platform for Delivering Intensified Substance Abuse Counseling," *Journal of Substance Abuse Treatment*, Vol. 36, No. 3, April 2009, pp. 331–338.

Kola, Lola, "Global Mental Health and COVID-19," *Lancet Psychiatry*, Vol. 7, No. 8, August 2020, pp. 655–657.

Larsen, Christopher, "Coronavirus Pandemic Spurs Increase in Telemedicine," U.S. Army, April 29, 2020. As of September 7, 2021:
https://www.army.mil/article/235087/coronavirus_pandemic_spurs_increase_in_telemedicine

Lin, Andrew H., Bethany L. Welstead, Brittany L. Morey, C. Becket Mahnke, Jacob H. Cole, and Michael G. Johnston, "Return on Investment Analysis of Health Experts onLine at Portsmouth: A 2-Year Review of the Navy's Newest Teleconsultation System," *Military Medicine*, Vol. 182, Nos. 5–6, May 2017, pp. e1696–e1701.

Lindsay, Jan A., Sonora Hudson, Lindsey Martin, Julianna B. Hogan, Miryam Nessim, Lauren Graves, Jeanne Gabriele, and Donna White, "Implementing Video to Home to Increase Access to Evidence-Based Psychotherapy for Rural Veterans," *Journal of Technology in Behavioral Science*, Vol. 2, No. 3–4, December 2017, pp. 140–148.

Lovell, Karina, Debbie Cox, Gillian Haddock, Christopher Jones, David Raines, Rachel Garvey, Chris Roberts, and Sarah Hadley, "Telephone Administered Cognitive Behaviour Therapy for Treatment of Obsessive Compulsive Disorder: Randomised Controlled Non-Inferiority Trial," *BMJ*, Vol. 333, No. 7574, October 28, 2006, article 883.

Maheu, Marlene M., Kenneth P. Drude, Katherine M. Hertlein, Ruth Lipschutz, Karen Wall, and Donald M. Hilty, "An Interprofessional Framework for Telebehavioral Health Competencies," *Journal of Technology in Behavioral Science*, Vol. 2, Nos. 3–4, December 2017, pp. 190–210.

———, "Correction to: An Interprofessional Framework for Telebehavioral Health Competencies," *Journal of Technology in Behavioral Science*, Vol. 3, No. 2, June 2018, pp. 108–140.

McGinty, Emma E., Rachel Presskreischer, Hahrie Han, and Colleen L. Barry, "Psychological Distress and Loneliness Reported by US Adults in 2018 and April 2020," *JAMA Network Open*, Vol. 324, No. 1, June 3, 2020, pp. 93–94.

Meadows, Sarah O., Charles C. Engel, Rebecca L. Collins, Robin L. Beckman, Joshua Breslau, Erika Litvin Bloom, Michael Stephen Dunbar, Marylou Gilbert, David Grant, Jennifer Hawes-Dawson, et al., *2018 Department of Defense Health Related Behaviors Survey (HRBS): Results for the Active Component*, Santa Monica, Calif.: RAND Corporation, RR-4222-OSD, 2021. As of September 22, 2021:
https://www.rand.org/pubs/research_reports/RR4222.html

Mehrotra, Ateev, Michael E. Chernew, David Linetsky, Hilary Hatch, and David A. Cutler, "The Impact of the COVID-19 Pandemic on Outpatient Visits: A Rebound Emerges," Commonwealth Fund, May 19, 2020a. As of September 7, 2021:
https://www.commonwealthfund.org/publications/2020/apr/impact-covid-19-outpatient-visits

———, "The Impact of the COVID-19 Pandemic on Outpatient Visits: Practices Are Adapting to the New Normal," Commonwealth Fund, June 25, 2020b. As of September 7, 2021:
https://www.commonwealthfund.org/publications/2020/jun/impact-covid-19-pandemic-outpatient-visits-practices-adapting-new-normal

Mehrotra, Ateev, Michael E. Chernew, David Linetsky, Hilary Hatch, David A. Cutler, and Eric C. Schneider, "The Impact of the COVID-19 Pandemic on Outpatient Care: Visits Return to Prepandemic Levels, but Not for All Providers and Patients," Commonwealth Fund, October 15, 2020c. As of September 7, 2021:
https://www.commonwealthfund.org/publications/2020/oct/impact-covid-19-pandemic-outpatient-care-visits-return-prepandemic-levels

MHS—*See* Military Health System.

Military Health System, "Telehealth Program," webpage, undated. As of September 7, 2021:
https://health.mil/Military-Health-Topics/Technology/Connected-Health/Telehealth-Program

Military Health System Communications Office, "MTFs Respond to COVID-19 with Increased Telehealth, Drive-Thrus," December 29, 2020. As of September 7, 2021:
https://www.health.mil/News/Articles/2020/12/29/MTFs-respond-to-COVID-19-with-increased-telehealth-drive-thrus

——, "MTF Facilities, Markets Set to Resume Transition Heading into 2021," January 6, 2021. As of September 7, 2021:
https://health.mil/News/Articles/2021/01/06/MTF-facilities-markets-set-to-resume-transition-heading-into-2021

Mohr, David C., Joyce Ho, Jenna Duffecy, Douglas Reifler, Leslie Sokol, Michelle Nicole Burns, Ling Jin, and Juned Siddique, "Effect of Telephone-Administered vs Face-to-Face Cognitive Behavioral Therapy on Adherence to Therapy and Depression Outcomes Among Primary Care Patients: A Randomized Trial," *JAMA*, Vol. 307, No. 21, June 6, 2012, pp. 2278–2285.

Morland, Leslie A., Carolyn J. Greene, Craig S. Rosen, Eric Kuhn, Julia Hoffman, and Denise M. Sloan, "Telehealth and eHealth Interventions for Posttraumatic Stress Disorder," *Current Opinion in Psychology*, Vol. 14, April 2017, pp. 102–108.

Morland, Leslie A., Stephanie Y. Wells, Lisa H. Glassman, Carolyn J. Greene, Julia E. Hoffman, and Craig S. Rosen, "Advances in PTSD Treatment Delivery: Review of Findings and Clinical Considerations for the Use of Telehealth Interventions for PTSD," *Current Treatment Options in Psychiatry*, Vol. 7, No. 3, September 2020, pp. 221–241.

Office of the National Coordinator for Health Information Technology, "What Are the Technical Infrastructure Requirements of Telehealth?" webpage, September 10, 2019. As of September 7, 2021:
https://www.healthit.gov/faq/what-are-technical-infrastructure-requirements-telehealth

Pamplin, Jeremy C., Konrad L. Davis, Jennifer Mbuthia, Steven Cain, Sean J. Hipp, Daniel J. Yourk, Christopher J. Colombo, and Ron Poropatich, "Military Telehealth: A Model for Delivering Expertise to the Point of Need in Austere and Operational Environments," *Health Affairs (Millwood)*, Vol. 38, No. 8, August 2019, pp. 1386–1392.

Pierce, Bradford S., Paul B. Perrin, Carmen M. Tyler, Grace B. McKee, and Jack D. Watson, "The COVID-19 Telepsychology Revolution: A National Study of Pandemic-Based Changes in U.S. Mental Health Care Delivery," *American Psychologist*, Vol. 76, No. 1, 2021, pp. 14–25.

Pineau, Gilles, Khalil Moqadem, Carole St-Hilaire, Robert Perreault, Éric Levac, and Bruno Hamel, *Telehealth: Clinical Guidelines and Technological Standards for Telepsychiatry, Summary*, Montreal, Quebec: Agence d'Évaluation des Technologies et des Modes d'Intervention en Santé, AETMIS 06-01, January 2006.

Place, Ronald J., Defense Health Agency, "Tiered Telehealth Health Care Support for COVID-19," memorandum to market directors, Falls Church, Va., March 27, 2020.

Pollard, Michael S., Joan S. Tucker, and Harold D. Green, Jr., "Changes in Adult Alcohol Use and Consequences During the COVID-19 Pandemic in the US," *JAMA Network Open*, Vol. 3, No. 9, September 29, 2020, article e2022942.

Public Law 114-328, National Defense Authorization Act for Fiscal Year 2017, December 23, 2016.

Public Law 116-92, National Defense Authorization Act for Fiscal Year 2020, December 20, 2019.

Rendle, Katharine A., Corey M. Abramson, Sarah B. Garrett, Meghan C. Halley, and Daniel Dohan, "Beyond Exploratory: A Tailored Framework for Designing and Assessing Qualitative Health Research," *BMJ Open*, Vol. 9, No. 8, August 27, 2019, article e030123.

Rosen, Craig S., Leslie A. Morland, Lisa H. Glassman, Brian P. Marx, Kendra Weaver, Clifford A. Smith, Stacey Pollack, and Paula P. Schnurr, "Virtual Mental Health Care in the Veterans Health Administration's Immediate Response to Coronavirus Disease–19," *American Psychologist*, Vol. 76, No. 1, January 2021, pp. 26–38.

Ryan, Gery W., and H. Russell Bernard, *Techniques to Identify Themes in Qualitative Data*, 2nd ed., Thousand Oaks, Calif.: Sage, 2000.

Santa Ana, Elizabeth J., Deidre L. Stallings, Bruce J. Rounsaville, and Steve Martino, "Development of an In-Home Telehealth Program for Outpatient Veterans with Substance Use Disorders," *Psychological Services*, Vol. 10, No. 3, August 2013, pp. 304–314.

Stoyanov, Stoyan R., Leanne Hides, David J. Kavanagh, Oksana Zelenko, Dian Tjondronegoro, and Madhavan Mani, "Mobile App Rating Scale: A New Tool for Assessing the Quality of Health Mobile Apps," *JMIR mHealth and uHealth*, Vol. 3, No. 1, March 2015, article e27.

Strong, Jessica, Jennifer Akin, and Drew Brazer, *Pain Points Poll Deep Dive: Understanding the Impact of COVID-19 on Mental Health*, Encinitas, Calif.: Blue Star Families, 2020. As of September 7, 2021:
https://bluestarfam.org/wp-content/uploads/2020/08/BSF-COVID-PPP-DeepDive-MentalHealth_ver2.pdf

TRICARE, "TRICARE Revises Telehealth Policy to Respond to COVID-19," updated June 23, 2020a. As of September 7, 2021: https://www.tricare.mil/CoveredServices/BenefitUpdates/Archives/05_18_2020_TRICARE_Revises_Telehealth_Policy_to_Respond_to_COVID_19

———, "New Telemental Health Services Available Through Telemynd," December 11, 2020b. As of September 7, 2021: https://www.hnfs.com/content/hnfs/home/tw/bene/res/beneficiary_news/new-telemental-health-services-available-through-telemynd.html

———, "Doctor on Demand Now Available to the TRICARE West Region," January 15, 2021. As of September 7, 2021: https://www.tricare-west.com/content/hnfs/home/tw/bene/res/beneficiary_news/doctor-on-demand-now-available-to-the-tricare-west-region.html

Tsiouris, Kostas M., Dimitrios Gatsios, Vassilios Tsakanikas, Athanasios A. Pardalis, Ioannis Kouris, Thelma Androutsou, Marilena Tarousi, Natasa Vujnovic Sedlar, Iason Somarakis, Fariba Mostajeran, et al., "Designing Interoperable Telehealth Platforms: Bridging IoT Devices with Cloud Infrastructures," *Enterprise Information Systems*, Vol. 14, No. 8, 2020, pp. 1194–1218.

Turgoose, David, Rachel Ashwick, and Dominic Murphy, "Systematic Review of Lessons Learned from Delivering Tele-Therapy to Veterans with Post-Traumatic Stress Disorder," *Journal of Telemedicine and Telecare*, Vol. 24, No. 9, October 2018, pp. 575–585.

U.S. Department of Defense, *Report to Armed Services Committees of the Senate and House of Representatives: Section 729 of the National Defense Authorization Act for Fiscal Year 2016 (Public Law 114-92), Plan for Development of Procedures to Measure Data on Mental Health Care Provided by the Department of Defense*, Washington, D.C., September 2016.

———, *Technology Solutions for Psychological Health: Report in Response to House Report 115-219, Pages 287–289 to Accompany H.R. 3219, the Department of Defense Appropriations Bill, 2018*, Washington, D.C., February 2019.

U.S. Department of Veterans Affairs, Office of Public and Intergovernmental Affairs, "VA Expands Access to Telehealth Services During COVID-19 Pandemic for Older, Rural and Homeless Veterans," press release, Washington, D.C., January 6, 2021. As of September 7, 2021: https://www.va.gov/opa/pressrel/pressrelease.cfm?id=5600

Uscher-Pines, Lori, James Thompson, Prentiss Taylor, Kristin Dean, Tony Yuan, Ian Tong, and Ateev Mehrotra, "Where Virtual Care Was Already a Reality: Experiences of a Nationwide Telehealth Service Provider During the COVID-19 Pandemic," *Journal of Medical Internet Research*, Vol. 22, No. 12, December 2020, article e22727.

VA—*See* U.S. Department of Veterans Affairs.

Varker, Tracey, Rachel M. Brand, Janine Ward, Sonia Terhaag, and Andrea Phelps, "Efficacy of Synchronous Telepsychology Interventions for People with Anxiety, Depression, Posttraumatic Stress Disorder, and Adjustment Disorder: A Rapid Evidence Assessment," *Psychological Services*, Vol. 16, No. 4, November 2019, pp. 621–635.

Waibel, Kirk H., Steven M. Cain, Todd E. Hall, and Ronald S. Keen, "Multispecialty Synchronous Telehealth Utilization and Patient Satisfaction Within Regional Health Command Europe: A Readiness and Recapture System for Health," *Military Medicine*, Vol. 182, No. 7, July 2017, pp. e1693–e1697.

Waltman, Scott H., Julie M. Landry, Lynette A. Pujol, and Bret A. Moore, "Delivering Evidence-Based Practices via Telepsychology: Illustrative Case Series from Military Treatment Facilities," *Professional Psychology: Research and Practice*, Vol. 51, No. 3, January 2020, pp. 205–213.

Webster, Paul, "Virtual Health Care in the Era of COVID-19," *The Lancet*, Vol. 395, No. 10231, April 11, 2020, pp. 1180–1181.

Zhang, Jonathan, Matt Boden, and Jodie Trafton, "Mental Health Treatment and the Role of Tele-Mental Health at the Veterans Health Administration During the COVID-19 Pandemic," *Psychological Services*, April 8, 2021.